Spectrum Natur  of
healthy oils and condiment e of
America's foremost nutriti
updated *Beyond Pritikin*. T
healthful essential fats and ing
weight loss, longevity, and good health.

SOME OF THE MEDICALLY
PROVEN BENEFITS
OF ESSENTIAL FAT . . .

WEIGHT LOSS
Essential fat helps to increase metabolic rate and energy production.
Easy weight loss is accomplished without strenuous dieting because
of balanced blood sugar and the elimination of food cravings.

HEART DISEASE
Essential fat lowers serum cholesterol triglycerides and regulates
blood pressure. It reduces the risk of thrombosis.

CANCER
Essential fat inhibits some types of cancer cell growth.

IMMUNE SYSTEM
Essential fat enhances the functioning of the T-suppressor
lymphocytes, which defend the body from invading bacteria and
viruses.

Spectrum Naturals thought you'd like to know.
For more information about healthy oils and fat:
Call our Consumer Voice Mail — 800 995 2705
Contact us by E-mail—spectrumnaturals@netdex.com

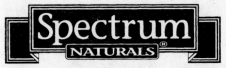

Petaluma, California

Beyond Pritikin

A Total
Nutrition Program
for Rapid Weight Loss,
Longevity,
and Good Health

Ann Louise Gittleman, M.S.
Certified Nutrition Specialist

COMPLETELY REVISED AND UPDATED

BANTAM BOOKS
NEW YORK · TORONTO · LONDON · SYDNEY · AUCKLAND

BEYOND PRITIKIN

A Bantam Book

PUBLISHING HISTORY
Bantam hardcover edition / April 1988
Bantam paperback edition / March 1989
Bantam revised edition / February 1996

Grateful acknowledgment is made for permission to reprint the following: Charts from the Nutrition Action Health letter, *copyright © 1985, Center for Science in the Public Interest. Excerpts from "Guess What's Coming To Dinner," copyright © 1987, Center for Science in the Public Interest. Excerpt from* Food Is Your Best Medicine *by Henry G. Bieler, M.D. Reprinted by permission of Random House, Inc.*

ISBN-13: 978-0-553-57400-5

ISBN-10: 0-553-57400-0

Published simultaneously in the United States and Canada

Bantam Books are published by Bantam Books, a division of Bantam Doubleday Dell Publishing Group, Inc. Its trademark, consisting of the words "Bantam Books" and the portrayal of a rooster, is Registered in U.S. Patent and Trademark Office and in other countries. Marca Registrada. Bantam Books, 1540 Broadway, New York, New York 10036.

PRINTED IN THE UNITED STATES OF AMERICA

OPM   19 18 17 16 15 14 13 12 11 10

This book is dedicated to
the memory of Harry Oliphant.

Revised Edition
Acknowledgments

Many thanks for the invaluable assistance from Jade Beutler, Rees Moerman, Melissa Diane Smith, and Neil Blomquist; biochemical guidance from Dallas Clouatre, Ph.D.; editorial guidance from Brian Tart; and the consistent support through the years from such great ladies as Ann Oliphant, Marcia Smith, Gracie Aldworth, Beth Hin, Anne Ross, Susan Meredith, Jane Heimlich, Valerie Diker, Joan Hamburg, Jinger Heath, Gloria Bein, Joanie Greggains, and my mother, Edith Gittleman. And, of course, my superman, James. I am especially appreciative of the hundreds of letters I have received from physicians, nutritionists, and readers who have been helped in some way by the information in *Beyond Pritikin*. Bless you all and bless the memory of my beloved cousin Gail Hersh Fannon, a devotee of health and nutrition who would have been very proud and excited about this book.

CONTENTS

Foreword by Dr. Julian Whitaker • xv
Preface to the 1996 Edition • xvii

1 Curbing Those Crazy Carbohydrates • 1

Glycemic Index • 8

2 Extending the Pritikin Prescription • 13

The Heart of the Matter • 14
Omega-3 and Omega-6 • 14
How Omega-3 and Omega-6 Work:
    The Prostaglandins • 16
The Essential Fats • 16
The Essential Fat Solution • 17
Looking Forward • 19

3 Pritikin Promises and Pitfalls • 21

The Diet/Disease Connection • 22
The Downside of the Pritikin Prescription • 23
Dietary Imbalances: Gluten Sensitivities and
    Candida Albicans • 23
New Findings: It's in the Fat • 27
Eat Fat and Lose Weight • 29
The Fat to Keep You Thin • 30
The Solution • 31

4 All About Essential Fats • 35

Basic Fat Groups • 36
How Fats Work in the Body • 38
The Infamous Four • 40
The Heat Factor • 40
The Hydrogenation Factor • 41
The Oxygen Factor • 41
The Homogenization Factor • 42

5 The *Beyond Pritikin* Diet Weight Loss Connection • 45

Brown Fat • 48
The Big Picture • 50

6 The *Beyond Pritikin* Diet Prostaglandin Protection • 52

The Benefits of Prostaglandins • 54

7 Polyunsaturates: Good Fats Gone Bad • 58

What Are the Essential Fats? • 60
Margarine: From Bad to Worse • 61

8 The Monounsaturates and Saturates Among Us • 66

The Monounsaturates • 66
Enter Canola Oil • 67
The Saturates • 68
The French Paradox • 69
Fast Foods • 69

Convenience Foods • 74
Is There a Solution? • 75

9 Cholesterol and the *Beyond Pritikin* Diet • 77

High-Density Lipoproteins (HDL) and Low-Density
    Lipoproteins (LDL) • 79
Triglycerides • 85

10 The *Beyond Pritikin* Diet Food Choices: Where the Essential Fats Are Found • 87

The GLA Fat Burners • 88
Omega-3s • 88
Essential Fat Dietary Supplements • 91
Caveat Emptor: What the Buyer Should Know
    About Fish Oil Capsules • 91
Additional Fat Fighters • 93
Cell Defense • 93
Garlic and Onions • 94

11 Fat-Burning Nutrients • 97

The Chromium Connection • 98
L-Carnitine • 99
Choline and Inositol • 100
Lipase to the Rescue • 101
Herbal Magic • 102

12 The Lowdown on Fiber • 103

13 New Light on Fitness • 108

14 Chemistry in the Kitchen • 113

Prime Contenders • 113
Prime Offenders • 115
Nutritional Bombshells • 116
The Life in Your Food • 117
Food Follies • 117
Nutritional Savvy • 118
Temperature Control • 119
Other Helpful Hints • 121
Selection of Vegetables and Fruits • 121
Successful Vegetable Storage • 122
Successful Fruit Storage • 123
Vegetable Preparation and Cooking • 124
Fruit Preparation and Cooking • 124
Fish, Fowl and Meat • 125
Successful Meat Storage • 126
Help Line • 126
Shellfish • 126
Seeds, Peanuts, Nuts, Beans, Egg Whites and
    Potatoes • 127
Desirable Cooking Methods • 127
Undesirable Cooking Methods • 129
Essential Utensils • 131
Essential Utensil Alert • 132

**15 The *Beyond Pritikin* Diet Master
Strategy • 135**

Finding Fat • 135
Sorting Out Salt • 136
The Yeast Problem:
    The Twentieth Century Epidemic • 137
Sweet Surrender • 138

Where to Shop • 138
Before You Take a Bite • 139
Food Combinations • 139
Stocking and Storing the Staples • 141
A Cleansing Formula • 149
Mail Order Suppliers of Organic Food • 151
A Note About Irradiated Food • 160

16 About the Diet: Questions and Answers • 162

The Eleven-Point Prescription • 170

17 The Two-Week Fat Flush • 172

Give Your Liver a Vacation • 173
The Fat Flush Program • 173
Detox While Dieting • 176
The Water Connection • 176
Putting It All Together • 177
Seasonal Tune-up • 179

18 The *Beyond Pritikin* Diet Prescription • 180

The *Beyond Pritikin* Diet Master Formula • 180
21-Day Master Menu Plan • 182
Recipes:
   Salad Dressings and Sauces • 191
   Pâtés • 196
   Soups • 198
   Main Events • 202
   Vegetables • 211
   Sweet Delights • 217

Nouvelle Puddings • 220
Fruit Gelatins • 221
Fresh Fruit Sorbets • 223
Grain Creations • 223
Food Equivalents • 224
Ten Transitional Tips • 231

19 Spices and Herbs of Life • 233

Herbal Magic • 233
Seasoning Savvy • 234
Spice It Up • 236

20 Eating Out Smart • 237

Where's the Beef? • 238
Small Plates • 239
Beyond Pritikin Ethnic Eating • 239
Safe Flying • 241
Cruising Cuisine • 241
Managing Margarine • 242

Appendix/Nutrition Education Resources • 243
References • 249
Recipe Index • 259
Index • 261

FOREWORD

In 1976, as a very young physician, I worked on the staff of the Pritikin Longevity Center, which was under the direction of its founder, Nathan Pritikin. This experience changed the course of my medical career. While I was there, I saw patients with severe degenerative diseases get well because of a simple but dramatic change in their diet that drastically reduced fat intake. The message from Pritikin and his famous Longevity Center was that fats are the primary cause of most of our serious and deadliest diseases, starting with heart disease and encompassing cancer, diabetes, high blood pressure, and obesity.

This message, however, is not totally accurate. The latest research has shown that fats, per se, are not the problem; it is the inappropriate types and excessive amounts of fat we consume that constitutes the problem. In fact, as is stated clearly throughout this book, certain fats are not only acceptable, but absolutely essential for optimal health.

Ann Louise Gittleman has done a masterful job maintaining the integrity of the original message of Nathan Pritikin's Longevity Center to reduce total fat intake, especially animal fats, while resurrecting the importance of the Omega-3 and Omega-6 fatty acids. These essential fatty acids, which cannot be manufactured in the body, are the precursors of the prostaglandins, some of the most fascinating, elusive, and potentially beneficial hormones. Using the Omega-3 and Omega-6 fatty acids that are found in certain foods, as well as supplements, to stimulate beneficial prostaglandin production is a natural and essential second step to the overall concept of fat reduction. Just as you cannot malign water because in certain situations it has the capacity to drown and kill, we should not malign fats because inappropriate and excessive intake creates illness.

Ms. Gittleman has done us all a service by showing us how the essential fats can and should be used in an overall program for living longer, losing weight, and reaching optimal health.

JULIAN WHITAKER, M.D.
Whitaker Wellness Institute

PROOF POSITIVE OF THE NEED FOR *BEYOND PRITIKIN*

A newly revised *Beyond Pritikin* is here thanks to all of you. As one devoted reader wrote in a letter to me: "*Beyond Pritikin* was so ahead of its time. Many of the trends you warned us about (how low-fat can make you fat, the carbohydrate overload consequences, how margarine is a health hazard, and the widespread effect of essential fat deficiency) are making headlines every day. Now that the public has caught up with your message, tell us more." And so, here is more.

The sad truth is that Americans are getting fatter. Fat phobia has overtaken the land, despite the lower-fat, lower-cholesterol diets. In fact, even though Americans have reduced their total fat intake from 37 percent to 34 percent during the last decade, our battle against the bulge is going in the wrong direction. In 1990, as part of its Healthy People 2000 Goals, the U.S. Department of Health set a goal of reducing the percentage of overweight Americans from 25 percent to 20 percent by the turn of the century. However, the most recent statistics show that if current trends continue, Americans not only will not reach that goal, but we will be farther from it than ever before. The latest National Health and Nutrition Exam Survey reported that, as a country, we have become 30 percent more overweight in the last decade. A University of Alabama at Birmingham report found that within a recent seven-year time frame young adults between the ages of 25 and 30 have gained an average of 10 pounds.

You know our war against being overweight has become big-time news when the cover page of the January 16, 1995, issue of *Time* magazine says in bold print: "Girth of a Nation" and tells us: "Here's some news that's hard to swallow: Despite the health craze, Americans are fatter than ever." Although it addressed a very important national issue, the article did not cover key reasons behind America's weight problems: the lack of essential fats in our diet, our increasing consumption of carbohydrates, and the connection between insulin and obesity. This book provides information about these frequently ignored but very important nutrition concepts.

Not only are many well-intentioned individuals gaining weight since the fat-free 1980s, they are now complaining of additional problems, such as fatigue, bloating, mood swings, and uncontrollable sugar cravings. These problems seem to be occurring in epidemic proportions since our nutritional leaders and our government have been encouraging us to eat low-fat, high-carbohydrate diets.

A new chapter in this book entitled "Curbing Those Crazy Carbohydrates" explains many of the reasons why Americans are getting heavier. In this chapter, I share some insights into the overlooked but far-reaching insulin effects of eating so many carbohydrates, even the complex ones. You will be introduced to the Glycemic Index, which lists carbohydrate-rich foods and measures the rate at which carbohydrates break down and release glucose into the body. You will learn that insulin is a fat-storage hormone par excellence, and the more pasta, bread, potatoes, and brown rice you eat, the more insulin your body will produce unless you balance those carbohydrates with some protein and fat. Too many carbohydrates eaten by themselves or without a sufficient balance of protein, fat, or exercise will stimulate the body to make and store fat and can cause other serious health problems.

In the new chapter "Fat-Burning Nutrients" you will learn why supplementing the diet with chromium, L-Carnitine (an amino acid), inositol, choline, and the enzyme lipase can enhance fat loss. For many individuals, these nutrients may provide a missing link to losing weight once and for all when combined with a good exercise regimen and a proper eating program.

I have revised the popular Two-Week Fat Flush by substituting flaxseed oil, one of the most promising and healthy Omega-3 oil sources, for the original expeller-pressed safflower oil. Buttery-tasting flaxseed oil is a real taste treat and is a health and beauty promoter as well. You will enjoy its taste in a brand-new, quick-and-easy recipe I have added called Perfect Pesto.

I think you will also be interested in reading about coconut oil, that so-called saturated fat villain used in most movie theaters for making popcorn. The new information I have included gives you some insights into food politics and the misinformation surrounding saturated fats. Also, many of the resource lists have been updated and the brand names on the shopping list have been completely revised.

I have modified almost every chapter to include the latest research findings and information that further substantiate the first edition. A case in point is the butter-versus-margarine debate. In the old edition, I discussed the health problems associated with margarine and its trans-fat accomplices such as vegetable shortening and processed vegetable oils. In May 1994, the *American Journal of Public Health* printed a commentary in which two Harvard researchers suggested that the trans-fatty acids found in margarine and in shortening may be linked to more than 30,000 heart disease deaths a year. Because of this and other similar health concerns, I have purposefully left intact many of my earlier observations and information that were right on track, as you will see.

More so than any other nutritionist in the country, I had the opportunity to witness firsthand the benefits and deficits of the low-fat diet when it first appeared and I wrote about them in the first edition of this book. Of the many readers who have thanked me for bringing this information to light, one especially moving thank-you came from brigadier general and former ophthalmologist Dr. Roland Pritikin, a very distant relative of the late Nathan Pritikin, who told me he bought several copies of *Beyond Pritikin* for his descendants. He said that every great invention or idea can always benefit from refinement, and I was touched to hear that he feels I have expanded upon the Pritikin-type, low-fat diet in a very positive way.

Essential fatty acids really are the most important health discovery in years. The 1990s are clearly evolving as the decade of the essential fatty acid revolution. As a nation, we must turn our attention to increasing the essential fats that will in turn regulate and balance both saturated fats and cholesterol.

It is very important to understand that certain types of fatty acids (which make up fats) and certain amino acids (which make up protein) are crucial for health and cannot be synthesized by the body. That means these nutrients need to be derived from food. However, there is no such thing as an essential carbohydrate. Keeping this in mind, the more you load up on carbohydrates and avoid fat and protein, the less you give your body the very nutrients it needs for its optimum health.

The more Americans continue to follow the low-fat, high-carbohydrate guidelines, the more we will continue to develop the very health problems we are trying to avoid. As current statistics show, cutting fat and eating mostly carbohydrates is not the complete answer. Now more than ever, we all need to understand the crucial concepts and facts about essential fatty acids I covered in the first edition of this book and which I have expanded upon in this edition. By including essential fats in our diets, we will enjoy lasting weight loss, longevity, and good health for tomorrow.

1

CURBING THOSE CRAZY CARBOHYDRATES

I know it is almost sacrilegious to criticize carbohydrates, but in light of so many negative effects from their imbalanced and excessive consumption, the time has come to take the carbohydrate craze to task. I am very concerned about the carbohydrate-related health problems so many of my clients are complaining about. Carbohydrate overloading tends to displace protein foods that the body needs for immunity, even blood sugar levels, proper hormonal functioning, and tissue repair. Plus the carbohydrates that everyone is eating, such as bread, pasta, and potatoes, are deficient in the essential fatty acids that control the cardiovascular, reproductive, and nervous systems. As a result, my clients are suffering from sugar cravings; lack of mental concentration; lack of energy; aging skin, hair, and nails; fluid retention; high triglycerides; weight problems; and the need for more and more sleep.

I realize carbohydrates are considered the preferred and cleanest-burning fuel source for human beings. But our national obsession with cutting the fat has produced a number of diet plans (for example, Dean Ornish's, John McDougall's, and Susan Powter's) that are unusually high in carbohydrates and, therefore, deficient in essential fatty acids—which ultimately are the real keys to overall health. As fat expert Edward Siguel, M.D., Ph.D. points out, even the U.S. Department of Agriculture's "Food Guide Pyramid" recommends that each day you eat from 6 to 11 servings of bread, cereal, rice, and potatoes—all foods that contain practically no essential fatty acids. Furthermore, if you decided to follow the government's guidelines, you would consume fats and oils sparingly because, according to the USDA, these foods contribute basically only calories to the diet.

I had a glimpse of carbohydrate-related health concerns (such as gluten intolerance and yeast overgrowth) in my early years working at the Pritikin Longevity Center. I discuss those conditions in the chapter entitled "Pritikin Promises and Pitfalls" and now expand upon them with some new observations. Of all the low-fat, high–complex-carbohydrate diets on the market today, the Pritikin Eating Plan is probably the most well balanced and researched. There also have been efforts made by the Pritikin educators to alert participants to the "glycemic" or blood sugar effect of certain carbohydrates (which I discuss later in this chapter), an issue that I feel is of vital importance.

Yet what I saw in those early years is nothing compared to the extreme diet histories my clients are manifesting now that they have become so fat-phobic. Many individuals are cutting down on basic nutritional staples such as eggs, meat, and butter due to misguided concerns about cholesterol and fat. Unfortunately, they have been substituting sugar for the missing fat and protein calories. What is showing up on diet histories now are record numbers of fat-free jelly beans, honey- or fruit juice–sweetened cookies, and low-fat (but sugar-rich) frozen yogurt.

All studies show that Americans are eating less fat today. The U.S. Department of Agriculture has reported a 14-pound drop in red meat consumption between 1980 and 1990. In the past 20 years, butter intake has dropped by a whopping 25 percent. But at the same time, the per capita ingestion of sugar has increased by 20 pounds per person per year. Those overweight have hit record numbers not because of increased fat intake but because Americans are overdoing the sugar and carbohydrates, which can, of course, turn to fat.

The popular diet mantras of "Eat more, weigh less" and "Stop the insanity" convey the faulty message that you can eat whatever you want, whenever you want, as long as the food is fat-free and full of fiber. Even the government has climbed on the "all fat is bad" bandwagon with the publication of the "Food Guide Pyramid." According to the Food and Drug Administration's new food labeling guidelines, in an average 2,000-calorie-a-day diet, more than half the calories should be from carbohydrates. (That's 300 grams a day!) Many diet gurus have joined the federal government and are now promoting a 70-percent carbohydrate diet. Consequently, there are a lot of people out there filling up on no-fat foods that contain up to 75 percent sugar.

So many people believe that nonfat means non-fattening that sales of no-fat and low-fat cookies have skyrocketed 70 percent during the last year, and the Number One cookie sold in America is no longer Oreos but fat-free SnackWells. But all those fat-free cookies and fat-free yogurts and muffins add up in carbohydrates and are usually loaded with sugar. Too much sugar can depress the immune system, feed yeast problems, and wreak havoc with blood sugar functioning. High sugar intake is linked to higher insulin levels, extreme hunger, and consequently, overeating and weight gain.

Speaking of high insulin levels, it seems that a growing number of Americans, maybe even 25 percent of all adults and an even larger percentage of the obese, have a problem with carbohydrate metabolism due to a resistance to insulin. Insulin is a hormone that metabolizes glucose from carbohydrates into energy. Insulin resistance is a condition in which body cells resist the action of insulin and the body overproduces insulin because of an excess of sugary and simple carbohydrate foods.

Fat phobia has spawned the carbohydrate craze that in turn has resulted in widespread insulin resistance and a whole new generation of carbohydrate addicts and carbohydrate sensitives. The term "carbohydrate addict" was first popularized by Mount Sinai Hospital researchers Drs. Richard and Rachel Heller in a book called *The Carbohydrate Addict's Diet* (Signet Books, 1993). The Hellers identified a disorder they called carbohydrate addiction and believe that nearly 75 percent of all overweight individuals may suffer from it. Individuals who have this condition have imbalanced insulin levels and are constantly hungry and crave carbohydrate-rich foods. In his book *Dr. Atkins' New Diet Revolution* (Evans, 1992), Robert Atkins, M.D., devotes an entire chapter, "Insulin—The Hormone That Makes You Fat," to insulin-related food cravings and weight problems.

Biochemist Barry Sears, Ph.D., has reported that high blood insulin levels promote fat storage and the inability to access stored fat because they activate the enzyme adipose tissue lipoprotein-lipase (AT-LPL). This enzyme acts like a master key to fat storage. Individuals who consistently eat foods that generate a high-insulin response, therefore, are promoting fat storage.

The term "carbohydrate toxicity" was coined by obesity specialist Dr. Wayne Calloway of George Washington University, who is equally critical of and concerned about carbohydrate preoccupation. In a *New York Times* article, he stated: "Chronic dieters often gain weight on high-carbohydrate diets because they have lost the ability to get rid of fluid."

The *New York Times* covered the completely ignored but very basic scientific information about the insulin connection to overweight conditions in its February 8, 1995, article entitled "So It May Be True After All: Eating Pasta Makes You Fat." The article quotes Dr. Artemis P. Simopoulos, former chairwoman of the nutritional coordinating committee of the National Institutes of Health and current president of the Center for Genetics Nutrition and Health in Washington. She said: "Insulin resistance is associated with obesity, and for many years it was thought to follow obesity. Today we know that in many cases, insulin resistance *precedes* obesity as well as some other diseases."

Obesity is just one of the many problems insulin resistance can cause. According to Dr. Gerald Reaven, a professor at the Stanford University Medical School who has studied insulin for three decades, insulin resistance is an underlying cause of a condition he calls "Syndrome X," which is associated with Type II diabetes, hypertension (high blood pressure), high triglyceride levels, and obesity. These, as many of you know, are some of the worst health problems Americans now face.

In my own work with thousands of clients, I have counseled many individuals with these same disastrous health problems after following excessively high-carbohydrate diets. I have had to convince them to limit their carbohydrate consumption and substitute more essential fatty acids and quality protein in their diets. Once I did, however, I have seen these individuals reverse dangerous heart disease risk factors and enjoy better health. I find it ironic that the people most apt to go on various versions of the recommended low-fat, high-carbohydrate diet are overweight, have high cholesterol levels, or have other heart disease risk factors. Unfortunately, many of them actually gain weight and increase their susceptibility to developing heart disease on such diets. Consider that while the death rate from heart disease has decreased (because of better intervention procedures such as angioplasty and bypasses), the incidence of heart disease has increased. Although America's total fat consumption has decreased and high-carbohydrate eating is on the rise, the number of cases of heart disease is not decreasing.

Even if you consistently eat only the complex carbohydrates, you may be setting the stage for fat buildup. Take

a good look at the following chart on page 8, known as
the Glycemic Index, which has been expanded upon and
adapted from the *Nutritional Manual of BioFoods, Inc.*, of
Santa Barbara, California. This chart was first developed
by David Jenkins, M.D., Ph.D., professor of medicine and
nutritional sciences at the University of Toronto. The list
is based upon measurements of real-life blood sugar levels after consumption of these foods. It lists a variety of
carbohydrate-rich foods and indicates the percentage
increase in blood sugar levels. Dr. Barry Sears is responsible for categorizing the list according to the varying
degrees of insulin production. As you can see, when
you consume mainly fat-free but high-glycemic foods
such as wheat bread, fruit juice, corn chips, and even
tofu ice cream, you may be fostering fat because the insulin these foods cause the body to release is a key fat-
promoting hormone.

So what can a weight-conscious person do?

I wish I had a magic carbohydrate formula that would
work for everyone all the time. The truth is we are all
very different and some people can tolerate more carbohydrates than others. Some individuals are slow oxidizers while others are fast. The slow oxidizer tends to
do better on a Pritikin-style diet (high carbohydrates—
with essential fatty acids, of course) while the fast oxidizer normally thrives on the Atkins-type diet (high
protein and fat). In *Your Body Knows Best* (Pocket Books,
1996) I discuss slow and fast oxidizers in greater detail.
What I can say for our purposes here is that, in general,
men seem to handle a greater carbohydrate load than
women. This is most likely because they have fewer fat
cells and more muscle mass, which makes their tissues
more metabolically active and, therefore, able to burn
up more carbohydrate calories. My female clients, however, seem to do better on a diet that ranges from 30 to
40 percent carbohydrates unless they are very physically
active. In this case, athletic women may be able to tolerate a diet closer to 50 to 55 percent carbohydrates.

Along with several top endocrinologists, I am becoming increasingly concerned about a growing number of ailments women and teenage girls develop when they load up on carbohydrates. These problems include obesity, acne, and a variety of hormonal imbalances including premenstrual syndrome, amenorrhea, excess facial hair, allergies, and sugar cravings. The more women embrace the high-carbohydrate style of eating, the more insulin is being secreted in their systems. Insulin causes the adrenal glands to produce androgens such as testosterone, which can prevent ovulation and wreak havoc with women's normal hormonal cycles.

In addition, high-carbohydrate consumption and lack of essential fats in our diets are contributing to the increasingly prevalent problem of *Candida albicans* (an overgrowth of yeast in the system that creates numerous digestive and reproductive symptoms), as well as hypothyroid conditions and adrenal insufficiency that can lead to food intolerances and sugar cravings. It is important to keep in mind that all of these conditions further depress the body's ability to metabolize carbohydrates. If you suffer from any of these conditions, it might be wise to monitor your carbohydrate intake more closely. Lack of zinc and chromium, both of which are insulin cofactors, can also impede carbohydrate metabolism. These minerals are grossly deficient in most Americans' diets due to food processing, poor food choices,and soil depletion.

What we can all do to be on the safe side is strive to keep insulin levels low. This is easily accomplished by eating meals that consist of a mixture of proteins, carbohydrates, and some fat. The good news about protein (such as fish, lean beef, lamb, eggs, poultry, and tempeh) is that it can increase metabolism by 30 percent, while a purely carbohydrate meal increases metabolism by only 10 percent. Protein also helps to balance insulin release through the production of a hormone called glucagon. Protein-induced glucagon in turn mobilizes fats from storage tissue, which helps weight loss. Glucagon acts in exactly the opposite way insulin does. By eating balanced meals, you get more steady blood sugar levels, and steady blood sugar leads to less hunger and the ability to burn stored body fat for safe, long-term weight loss.

Fats (such as butter, olive oil, sesame oil, and natural salad dressings) also slow down insulin release in the system. Plus, a little bit of fat goes a long way in making you feel full, so you won't be tempted to overeat. Besides, the essential fats (such as safflower oil and flaxseed oil) have metabolic-raising effects to boot. When you start replacing the right fat, most of you will be balancing your carbohydrate intake automatically.

The two eating plans in this book were developed not only to put fats back in their rightful dietary place, but also to take into account varying carbohydrate tolerances. The Two-Week Fat Flush is a low-carbohydrate diet designed primarily for cleansing as well as weight loss. This program is geared toward jump-starting your system and is more severe and stringent than the 21-Day Master Menu Plan. The 21-Day Master Menu Plan can also be used for weight loss—although it may be slower—but it does provide a higher carbohydrate intake, which may be more appropriate for some individuals. The basic menus can be followed for a maintenance program by adding even more carbohydrate portions (from cereal, bread, and starchy vegetables) until you find the amount that helps you look and feel your best. All of this is spelled out for you in the section entitled "The *Beyond Pritikin* Diet Prescription."

Glycemic Index

A. Rapid inducers of insulin

GLYCEMIC INDEX GREATER THAN 100%

Puffed Rice
Corn Flakes
Puffed Wheat

Maltose
French baguette
Millet
Instant white rice
40% Bran Flakes
Rice Krispies
Weetabix
Tofu ice cream substitute

GLYCEMIC INDEX = 100%

Glucose
White bread
Whole wheat bread

GLYCEMIC INDEX BETWEEN 90 AND 100%

Grape Nuts
Carrots
Parsnips
Barley (whole meal)
Muesli
Shredded Wheat
Apricots
Corn chips

GLYCEMIC INDEX BETWEEN 80 AND 90%

Rolled oats
Oat bran
Honey
White rice
Brown rice
Bananas
White potatoes
Corn
Rye (whole meal)
Shortbread
Ripe bananas

Ripe mangoes
Ripe papayas

GLYCEMIC INDEX BETWEEN 70 AND 80%

All-Bran
Kidney beans
Wheat (coarse)
Buckwheat
Oatmeal cookies

B. Moderate inducers of insulin

GLYCEMIC INDEX BETWEEN 60 and 70%

Raisins
Mars candy bar
Spaghetti (white)
Spaghetti (whole wheat)
Pinto beans
Macaroni
Rye (pumpernickel)
Bulgur
Couscous
Wheat kernels
Beets
Apple juice
Applesauce

GLYCEMIC INDEX BETWEEN 50 and 60%

Peas (frozen)
Sucrose
Potato chips
Yams
Barley
Custard
Dried white beans
Green bananas
Lactose

GLYCEMIC INDEX BETWEEN 40 and 50%

Sweet potatoes
Rye (whole grain)
Oatmeal (steel cut)
Sponge cake
Butter beans
Grapes
Oranges
Orange juice

GLYCEMIC INDEX BETWEEN 40 and 50%

Navy beans
Peas (dried)
Bran
Lima beans

C. Reduced insulin secretion

GLYCEMIC INDEX BETWEEN 30 and 40%

Apples
Black-eyed peas
Chickpeas
Ice cream
Milk (skim)
Milk (whole)
Yogurt
Tomato soup
Pears
Fish sticks (breaded)

GLYCEMIC INDEX BETWEEN 20 and 30%

Lentils
Fructose
Plums
Peaches

Grapefruit
Cherries

GLYCEMIC INDEX BETWEEN 10 and 20%

Soybeans
Peanuts

2

EXTENDING THE PRITIKIN PRESCRIPTION

Health is a journey, not a destination.
—ANONYMOUS

The Pritikin prescription for optimum health is a low-fat, low-cholesterol, low-sodium, high-complex-carbohydrate diet combined with regular aerobic exercise. In caloric percentages, Pritikin's diet is composed of 5 to 10 percent fat, 10 to 15 percent protein, and 80 percent complex carbohydrate. It consists of whole grains, beans, vegetables, fruits, nonfat dairy products, and small amounts of protein from beef, fowl, and fish. Protein consumption is limited to a lean 3.5 ounces a day in order to reduce total fat and cholesterol intake because most animal protein foods have high levels of fat and cholesterol.

Clearly a spartan diet, the Pritikin diet was successful in getting people off fat, salt, sugar, alcohol, coffee, and tobacco. It provided a firm foundation for sound and healthy eating habits. It promoted whole foods and regular daily exercise. In many cases the supervised program reduced blood pressure levels, decreased cholesterol levels, and greatly diminished insulin use by diabetics.

Although not a medical doctor, Pritikin was an avid

medical researcher. His particular interest was coronary heart disease, because in 1955 he was diagnosed as suffering from a severe heart condition. Convinced that there was a correlation between diet and health, for over twenty-five years Pritikin researched medical literature on the degenerative diseases of the Western world such as cardiovascular disease, high blood pressure, diabetes, and cancer. He also studied the dietary patterns and lifestyles of societies which had much lower rates of degenerative illness. Pritikin then modeled his diet after the basic high-starch (complex carbohydrate) and low-fat food patterns of primitive cultures such as the Tarahumara Indians of northwestern Mexico, the Bantus of South Africa, and the natives of New Guinea.

The Heart of the Matter

The heart of the Pritikin diet is its extremely low fat content. He based his low-fat emphasis on his research findings that high-fat, high-cholesterol diets are linked with degenerative disease in the developed nations. Medical literature suggests that saturated fat can raise serum cholesterol levels, and that serum cholesterol is a key factor in the incidence of heart disease—the nation's Number One killer. Pritikin, however, restricted not only the saturated fats (which usually come from meat and full-fat dairy products) but banned all fats, including the unsaturated fats from vegetable, nut, and seed sources. Pritikin didn't acknowledge the beneficial value of any fats in the diet.

Pritikin's review of diets from all over the world, obviously prejudiced by his personal health concern, focused on the therapeutic cardiovascular aspects. Yet his investigations missed crucial evidence about the role of fat in the diet.

Omega-3 and Omega-6

Pritikin's research somehow overlooked the revolutionary fat insights of researchers H. O. Bang and John Dyerberg presented in a 1978 study published in *Lancet,* the highly respected British medical journal. Drs. Bang and Dyerberg investigated the diet of native Greenland Eskimos. They reported that despite an extremely high-fat, high-cholesterol diet, the Eskimos have a very low incidence of coronary heart disease, diabetes, and cancer. The connection between the Eskimos' high-fish diet and their low heart disease rate was suspected as early as 1855. These early population studies resurfaced with the Bang and Dyerberg observations of the 1970s.

It was reported that the traditional Eskimo diet contains over 70 percent of its calories in fat, and yet the Eskimos are free of killer degenerative illness such as heart disease. This figure represents a far cry from the recommended 10 percent of fat calories suggested by Nathan Pritikin to prevent and control disease. Despite this important new information published in 1978, Pritikin writes in his 1979 book *The Pritikin Program for Diet and Exercise,* "We feel that fats are so bad for you that you should eat no more than 5 to 10 percent fat."

The key to the Eskimos' excellent health is the kind of fat they eat. Eskimos get their fat from marine life (seal, whale, walrus) and fatty cold-water fish (herring, mackerel and salmon) that make up most of their diet. These foods contain marine oils which are high in two important Omega-3 fatty acids called eicosapentaenoic acid, or EPA, and docosahexaenoic acid, or DHA. *Omega-3 fatty acids in the form of EPA and DHA have been shown to protect the cardiovascular system.*

In fact, as early as the 1970s Hoffman-LaRoche published clinical data that showed the positive effects of adding fat in the form of GLA to the diet.

Another acknowledged leader in fat research, Dr. David Horrobin, began publishing in the early 1980s. Horrobin reported outstanding health results with another kind of fat, evening primrose oil, which contains substantial amounts of an Omega-6 fatty acid called gamma linolenic acid, or GLA. He showed that GLA helped cardiovascular problems, weight loss, inflammatory diseases such as arthritis, disorders of the immune system, alcoholism, premenstrual syndrome, and skin, hair, and nail conditions.

How Omega-3 and Omega-6 Work: The Prostaglandins

The Omega-3 and Omega-6 fatty acids work together in the body by forming hormonelike substances called prostaglandins. The role of prostaglandins is to control the human body's daily function. As an indication of how important prostaglandins are, it is interesting to note that prostaglandin researchers were awarded three Nobel Prizes in medicine in 1982.

Prostaglandins control *all* body functions at the cellular level. They are vital in regulating the cardiovascular, reproductive, immune, and central nervous systems. Prostaglandins are needed to control clotting, inflammation, tumor growth, and allergies. The onset of disease is the result of a prostaglandin imbalance.

Prostaglandins protect against heart disease by:

- Making the blood thinner, less sticky, and less likely to clot
- Reducing platelet clumping
- Lessening constriction of the blood vessels

However, without a balance of both essential fat families, prostaglandins cannot perform their crucial and varied regulatory functions in the body.

The Essential Fats

There are two major types of essential fats: Omega-3 oils from flax and fish, and Omega-6 oils from plant and botanical sources such as natural vegetable oils, borage, and evening primrose oil. These two families of essential fatty acids perform two major roles: (1) they form the cell membrane that surrounds every cell in the body, and (2) they are the source of prostaglandins, which have far-reaching regulatory effects throughout the human body.

Now is the time to reinstate essential fats into our diet because of these reasons:

• The decades-long influence of the no- to low-fat, high-carbohydrate diet model (à la Pritikin, Ornish, McDougall, and Powter) with its exclusion of fats including healthful fats;

• Dietary trends toward eating fast foods in which the cooking process may make the fats harmful to the body; and,

• Misinformation and misleading propaganda about how indispensable the right fats are for total health.

The Essential Fat Solution

Essential fats are a fundamental component of what I call my *Beyond Pritikin* Diet. The Essential Fat Solution is based on three crucial points:

1. Essential fat is fat that is absolutely necessary for the regulation of every function in the human body.

2. Essential fat is fat that must be included in the diet because it cannot be manufactured by the body.

3. Essential fat is fat that has not been nutritionally altered from its natural state by food processing or faulty cooking practices, yet has been purified of oil-soluble pesticides and herbicide residue.

New findings about the role of good fats are reported almost daily from around the world. In 1994, a study was done by Boston University Medical Center. Dr. Edward Siguel suggested that the addition of essential fatty acids can eliminate heart disease risk. Siguel is not the first to say that our Number One killer is really symptomatic of this massive deficiency.

Believe it or not, almost 80 million Americans are too fat and yet fat deficient. Sounds like a contradiction, doesn't it? It is even more of a contradiction when you consider that nearly 40 percent of the calories in the standard American diet comes from fat.

The right kind and the right amount of fat will allow you to lose weight effortlessly and painlessly without becoming preoccupied with dieting. Fats provide long-term satiety. I have seen how zero-fat diets lead to persistent food cravings, continuous hunger, and overeating of calories (which, of course, turn to fat). Adding, not subtracting, enough of the healthy kind of fat to the diet is one of the easiest ways, in combination with exercise, to attain and maintain normal weight.

Obesity is only one of our national health problems that may be caused by lack of essential fat in the diet. As you will experience, essential fat is not only good for your waistline, it offers protection from many of the diseases that befall modern man. According to the studies of prominent fat researchers like Drs. William Connor, Donald Rudin, David Horrobin, Barry Sears, Udo Erasmus, and Edward Siguel, essential fat (from EPA-containing fish oils, and GLA-containing vegetable and botanical oils) has proven effective in controlling, preventing, and reversing a number of disease conditions.

Essential fat benefits:

WEIGHT LOSS

Essential fat helps to increase metabolic rate and energy production. Easy weight loss is accomplished without strenuous dieting because of balanced blood sugar and no more food cravings

HEART DISEASE

Essential fat lowers serum cholesterol and triglycerides, and regulates blood pressure. It reduces the risk of thrombosis.

CANCER

Essential fat inhibits some types of cancer cell growth.

DIABETES

Essential fat promotes more effective insulin utilization.

RHEUMATOID ARTHRITIS

Essential fat functions as an anti-inflammatory catalyst.

PREMENSTRUAL SYNDROME

Essential fat alleviates 90 percent of PMS tensions and discomfort.

IMMUNE SYSTEM

Essential fat enhances the functioning of the T-suppressor lymphocytes that defend the body from invading bacteria and viruses.

SKIN

Essential fat clears psoriasis, eczema, and acne.

NAILS

Essential fat hardens splitting, brittle nails.

CANDIDA ALBICANS

Essential fat controls yeast infections.

ALLERGIES

Essential fat aids in preventing allergic response.

Looking Forward

Nathan Pritikin was the first to really recognize that the standard American diet encouraged excessive intake of fat, but he did not distinguish between healthful fat and unhealthful fat and so excluded them all, including the fats from the Omega-3 and Omega-6 families, which are now recognized as absolutely crucial for health. Now there is a new generation of fat-free gurus, free-lance health writers, and dieticians who call for the banning of *all* fats. Fat phobia has even resulted in the nutritional travesty called the "Food Guide Pyramid" in which fats and oils are portrayed as providing "calories and little else nutritionally." The emphasis, ironically, on the bread, cereal, rice, and pasta group (6–11 servings) encourages excess starch consumption, which I believe is the main reason that obesity is on the rise, despite low-fat, low-cholesterol intake.

Beyond Pritikin is about looking forward and extending the basic foundation of the Pritikin diet to a diet that includes essential fat and a balanced carbohydrate intake—a life-supporting, lifelong eating plan based on state-of-the-art nutritional findings. That's why I call my program the *Beyond Pritikin* Diet. And since people eat food, not nutrition, my diet is based on a return to the pleasures of eating seasonally fresh, wholesome foods. Finally, understanding that certain fats can be good for you is a boon to the health-conscious cook and consumer. Fat goes a long way in making food more palatable because it is such a potent flavor carrier and enhancer. And as an added benefit to the weight-conscious reader, this eating program will also help you lose weight.

By eating the right carbohydrates, protein, and fats and feeling energetic once again, we will all be able to give thanks and remember something we have long forgotten in this era of fat phobia: It is a privilege to eat!

3

PRITIKIN PROMISES
AND PITFALLS

*Most maladies that afflict humanity result from bad food or
excess of food that may even have been wholesome.*
—MAIMONIDES, THIRTEENTH CENTURY

The year 1985 marked the end of the low-fat era and gave
birth to the philosophy that is the basis of the *Beyond
Pritikin* Diet. It was the year that Nathan Pritikin, the
champion of the fat-free diet, died. It was also the year
in which three landmark studies were published in the
prestigious *New England Journal of Medicine*. These
studies, from the Harvard Medical School, the Oregon
Health Sciences University, and the University of Leiden
in the Netherlands, correlated fish and the oil (fat) contained in fish with reducing cardiovascular disease and
possibly rheumatoid arthritis and asthma as well.

Pritikin himself was the herald for a new age in the
1970s and early '80s which captured the attention of the
American public. He advocated self-health in the form of
diet and exercise. More than any other diet spokesman,
he represented the fitness spirit of the times. The Pritikin
Longevity Centers pioneered the burgeoning health con-
sciousness and paved the way for the new breed of medical spas and preventive health centers that exist
throughout the country today.

The Diet/Disease Connection

Pritikin's 1974 book, *Live Longer Now*, provided the model in the years that followed for a whole series of government reports on dietary recommendations. His low-fat, high–complex-carbohydrate message was echoed in the 1977 *Dietary Goals for the United States* issued by the Senate Select Committee on Nutrition and Human Needs. Then, in 1979, came the *Surgeon General's Report on Health Promotion and Disease Prevention*, which said: *"You the individual can do more for your own health and well-being than any doctor, any hospital, any drug, any exotic medical advice."*

This simple yet significant statement from the U.S. Surgeon General represented a major step forward in the attitude of traditional medical practices. It shifted the responsibility for health from doctors, drugs, and surgery to the individual. The Pritikin program epitomized this self-care attitude from the beginning.

A final accolade to the Pritikin principles came in 1982, when the National Academy of Sciences published a major report which, for the first time, associated dietary patterns with certain forms of cancer. At long last, medical evidence had linked another killer disease, cancer, to diet. Health had become a personal responsibility, requiring lifestyle and dietary changes. Now those who were ready to take this responsibility were hungry for "diet" information.

At the Pritikin Center where I was Director of Nutrition, I witnessed dramatic improvements in many participants who followed Pritikin's diet and whose case histories later became the statistics supporting the Pritikin program. Every day I scanned medical charts and reviewed blood values that demonstrated Pritikin's claim that "cholesterol was lowered on the average a full 24 percent and that over 50 percent of the adult-onset diabetics leave virtually free of insulin and after two weeks most hypertensives leave drug-free with lowered blood pressure."

The Downside of the Pritikin Prescription

Slowly, however, I began to experience the downside of the Pritikin experience. Even though the participants at the Center demonstrated many positive changes while staying there, some complained of problems after leaving, or when they returned for refresher courses. There were complaints about weight gain, feeling hungry all the time no matter how much food was eaten, and problems because of the inordinate amount of time needed to prepare and eat six to eight small meals a day. I also noticed a rather curious phenomenon among those participants who were on the program from one to two years—the appearance of vertical ridges on the fingernails, a syndrome that signals a nutritional deficiency.

Dietary Imbalances: Gluten Sensitivities and *Candida Albicans*

I began to wonder about the potential shortcomings of the Pritikin program. Pritikin studied the diet of the Tarahumara Indians of northwestern Mexico as a model for his low-fat, high-starch regimen. The Tarahumaras are recognized as the greatest long-distance runners in the world. Their diet features corn as the staple, while a major emphasis in the Pritikin plan is on whole grains. While both corn and grains are classified as complex carbohydrates, they differ in one major respect: *Grains such as wheat, rye, oats, and barley contain a substance called gluten, to which many individuals are sensitive.*

It used to be thought that gluten intolerance, also called celiac or sprue disease, was a relatively rare occurrence affecting only a small number of people. But recent findings show that more and more people are unable to assimilate wheat and similar grains because of excessive consumption of these foods. What we are now seeing is that the minority is becoming a majority with minor gluten malabsorption. When the high-carbohydrate diets came in style, many individuals became over-enthusiastic with the amounts of whole grains they added to their diet. Grains for breakfast in the form of cereal, then in sandwiches for lunch, in pasta for dinner, and in whole-grain cookies and muffins for snacks, created a metabolic overload.

Gluten is the protein portion of the grain that gives dough its elastic consistency. When gluten-rich grains are eaten in excess, persistent intestinal gas, bloating, irregular bowel movements, and fatigue can occur. Diarrhea, anemia, pallor, and mental instability can be created by gluten intolerance.

There is a growing number of people who suffer from minor gluten malabsorption. Classic gluten intolerance occurs in 1 out of 25,000 people. I believe there is a subclinical problem, which has been going on since the high-carbohydrate diet became so stylish, with consuming whole grains morning, noon, and night. Most people are simply not aware that their digestive problems and lack of energy are caused by their excessively grain-rich diet.

Gluten intolerance has been linked to a number of disease conditions, such as multiple sclerosis, schizophrenia, arthritis, and autism. In adults, a kind of itching eczema characterized by small red bumps has been linked to gluten intolerance. This protein-containing substance found in grains impairs the intestinal lining and interferes with nutrient absorption. When the intestinal tract is diseased or damaged, the B vitamins—especially folic acid and B-12—are not well absorbed. Such deficiencies can result in classical anemia as well as mental confusion in addition to the primary gluten intolerance. Often vitamins or even vitamin injections are necessary to replace lost nutrients due to malabsorption.

In his book *Can a Gluten-Free Diet Help You . . . How?* (New Canaan, CT: Keats, 1992), Lloyd Rosenvold suggests that conditions as diverse as Down's syndrome, Alzheimer's, myasthenia gravis, and a whole host of associated autoimmune disorders may have their roots in gluten intolerance. Hypertension, depression, and psoriasis are also discussed and linked to gluten problems. Rosenvold refers to the work of Australian physician Chris Reading, who corroborates many of Rosenvold's findings.

The high fiber content of gluten-rich grains tends to carry minerals *out* of the body before they can be absorbed. Calcium, folic acid, and iron are often deficient in a heavy grain diet, as well as fat-soluble vitamins A and E. These combined vitamin and mineral deficiencies can create irregular menstrual cycles, vague aches and pains in the bones, and perhaps the ridged fingernail condition. Although the Pritikin diet is often referred to as the Caveman's Diet, the cavemen didn't eat grains. Cavemen relied on meats, vegetables, beans, fruits, berries, and nuts. Grains are relatively new foods to the human gut, having been around for only 10,000 years. I think that the rise in carbohydrate consumption can be traced to several trends over the past two decades. In 1971, *Diet for a Small Planet* was published. The author, Frances Moore Lappe, suggests that by combining grains with beans, protein values can be increased. As a result many readers became convinced that they could and indeed should eat more grains. The phenomenal growth of vegetarianism has further encouraged grain consumption. This movement has generated many national magazines (such as *Vegetarian Times* and *The Vegetarian Gourmet*) as well as many cookbooks that prominently feature whole grains. Pick up any women's magazine and you will be inundated with ways to make whole wheat and brown rice more exciting.

None of these magazines or cookbooks is concerned with possible gluten intolerance. Wheat is perhaps one of the most common foods people can be sensitive to and it is in everything—breads, pasta, cookies, cakes, and piecrust.

Thanks to my mentor, Nathan Pritikin, the real pioneer of the no- to low-fat diet trend that has exploded today, the image of the carbohydrate has been transformed. Once considered fattening and a symbol for the poor, pasta has become glamorous and is now *très chic*. Current diet wisdom suggests it is really all the butter and creamy sauces on your pastas that are the real problems. In fact, nowadays pasta is recommended for weight-restricted diets as well as for carbo loading for athletes.

Prominent books such as *The Carbohydrate Craver's Diet*, by Judith Wurtman of MIT, and Jane Brody's Good Food Book: *Living the High Carbohydrate Way*, by *New York Times* journalist Jane Brody, have touted the value of health-promoting starch foods like grains, beans, and potatoes. Plus the recent emphasis on the value of increasing dietary fiber in the form of whole grains to ward off colon cancer and constipation has resulted in overconsumption of cereals, grains, and flours.

A major problem in all of this carbohydrate overload is that gluten-containing grains are the predominant carbohydrate food that Americans are ingesting.

Which grains are gluten-free? Millet, corn, rice, quinoa, amaranth, and buckwheat. Flours made from arrowroot, tapioca, potatoes, and soybeans are good wheat-flour substitutes. (Some people can tolerate the ancient wheat grains spelt and kamut although they are not gluten free.) But restricting grain from the diet may not be the only dietary change that needs to be made. Often a lactose intolerance accompanies the inability to digest gluten. So, avoiding milk is in order. Milk products like cheese and yogurt can usually be tolerated.

The various restrictions of the Pritikin diet promoted the overuse not only of grains but of yeast-related foods. These include fermented foods such as soy sauce and oil-free vinegar dressings, mushrooms (from the fungus family), and yeast-containing breads and crackers. Tomato sauce, a popular element in the diet, is also yeast-related because its processing creates fermentation.

We know today through the writings of Drs. Orian Truss and William Crook, authorities on fungus-related illnesses, that these foods contribute to an internal condition called polysystemic chronic candidiasis—a disorder that is said to affect one out of three Americans. This condition, which comes about through extended use of antibiotics, cortisone, and birth control pills, is fed by yeast-related foods and a high-carbohydrate diet. *The fungus that contributes to disease states is called* Candida albicans *and may be the basis of allergies, depression, and various environmental sensitivities.*

Despite my concern about the dietary imbalances I began to observe, my days at the Pritikin Center were personally fulfilling when I considered the overall successes. Our work made a difference in people's lives who were now much more aware of the need to eat sensibly and exercise regularly. All the while, I kept abreast of the latest health and nutritional research from doctors, clinics, and journals from around the world. As a health researcher, I continually sought nutritional answers to new illnesses and disorders such as food and chemical reactions, premenstrual syndrome, and *Candida albicans.* These new disorders began to surface and became as problematic as the degenerative diseases (such as heart disease) that the Pritikin-style diets were created to alleviate. There now appears to be a whole new generation of twenty-first-century health invaders that the fat-free, high-carbo diet models weren't designed to address.

New Findings: It's in the Fat

I left Pritikin in 1982 to research the underlying causes of the newly discovered health invaders and incorporate the latest findings into the basic Pritikin prescription of diet and exercise. In search of more answers, I traveled to Europe to study the health techniques of different clinics. While the results in these clinics were impressive, the need for a practical way to enhance immunity and ward off disease was ignored.

Back in the United States, the most exciting research that surfaced identified certain kinds of fats with helping to control disease conditions:

• Fat from the Omega-3 fatty acid family found in fish oil was being used to treat heart disease, arthritis, migraines, and even cancer.

• GLA, an Omega-6 fatty acid found in certain botanical oils such as borage and evening primrose, was having great success in treating premenstrual syndrome, infertility, alcoholism, and immunity disorders.

While in the Pritikin view fat was the dietary cause of most degenerative disease, the latest medical opinion was that the *right* kind of fat was a panacea for most diseases.

Pritikin said fat was the problem. I was seeing fat as the solution.

I became more engrossed in the fat issue and found that *fat is one of the most basic yet least understood nutrients.* Pritikin was not wrong about the dangers of polyunsaturated fats when he wrote: "In several respects unsaturated fats may be worse for you than saturated fats." But he didn't differentiate between the commercially processed and natural varieties. Leading health organizations such as the American Heart Association suggest that saturates should be replaced with polyunsaturates, but they don't differentiate between the good and bad fats either. The matter of commercial processing of fat is crucial. It destroys the essential fatty acids, which become unusable and harmful to the human body.

As a professional food educator, I was concerned about how an indispensable food nutrient like fat could become so dispensable. During the course of my research, I found out that the real problem was not so much what fat was doing to us, but what we were doing to fat.

Primary Factors That Devitalize and Alter Fats

- heat
- hydrogenation
- oxidation
- homogenization

The fate of all fat is determined basically by these conditions. *These four factors can chemically change the most widely consumed fatty food sources into foods unsuitable for human consumption.* Commercial vegetable oil, margarine, and whole milk are prime examples of devitalized, even harmful foods because the fat content has been altered. The *Beyond Pritikin* Diet will show you how fat has become misrepresented and misunderstood because of the health-destroying effects of heat, oxidation, hydrogenation, and homogenization.

Eat Fat and Lose Weight

You will learn, as I did, that not all fats are bad. As a matter of fact, the right kind and the right amount of fat is essential for good health and lasting weight loss.

Weight loss? you say. That's right. Weight loss is a completely unexpected benefit of eating the right kind of fat. My female patients who started supplementing their diets with foods or food supplements high in certain kinds of fat began to report surprising weight loss results. These women were not dieting, per se, but were prescribed a special fat nutrient, GLA, to control their PMS problems, recurring yeast infections, and arthritis. One woman who had a weight problem called me to say that not only was she elated over her cramp-free menstrual period but that she had somehow lost weight, too. She exclaimed, "I can't get over the fact that I'm eating fat and losing weight!"

The difference, of course, was the *right* kind of fat. The standing joke among my patients was how Pritikin's former Director of Nutrition was now promoting fat—what I told them was called an essential fat. Truth is stranger than fiction, I guess, because that was exactly what was happening. Fat was the answer to many menstrual problems suffered by my clients. Furthermore, fat was in to stay thin.

The weight loss phenomenon of the *Beyond Pritikin* Diet became so popular in my private practice that I was getting referrals from clients who were encouraging their obese friends to see me. I had to find out what was really going on inside the body when the outside results were so dramatic.

I learned that *the right kind of fat—an essential fat— stimulates a mechanism in the body that in turn burns fat.* This internal fat burner is what scientists call *"brown fat."* Brown fat may well be the most important discovery to explain why some people can remain thin while eating everything in sight while others, no matter how restricted their caloric intake, still cannot lose weight. In the 1990s the concept of burning fat through certain thermogenic (metabolic-raising) products has become quite the rage. A basic theory behind the ingestion of certain "fat burners" (particularly vitamins, minerals, herbs, and amino acids) is that they help to reactivate brown adipose tissue, or brown fat (BAT), which is the fat-burning process identified below.

The Fat to Keep You Thin

There are basically two kinds of fat cells in the body: white fat and brown fat.

- *White fat is the insulating fat layer under the skin that stores excess calories as fat.*

- *Brown fat is a special fat-burning tissue that burns excess calories for heat rather than body energy.*

Most of what we know about brown fat has come from animal studies. Animals depend on their brown fat to keep them warm during hibernation. Brown fat alone generates one-fourth of the heat produced by all of the other body tissues combined. It apparently is a specially conditioned body warmer that operates when extra heat is needed.

Brown fat is located deeper in the body than white fat—in the thoracic area along the backbone and the back of the neck, and in the adrenal glands, kidneys, and aorta. The brown color is caused by the presence of concentrated fat-burning cellular units called mitochondria. The quest has been to find out what activates the mitochondria in the brown fat. What researchers discovered was that *thin people have "activated" brown fat, while overweight individuals have dormant brown fat.* Also, brown fat decreases with age, which may account for why many people gain weight as they grow older. Whatever the age, brown fat needs the right kind of "activator" so the body will burn, rather than store, more calories. A breakthrough came when it was discovered that GLA—gamma linolenic acid—a special fat nutrient, was shown to "activate" brown fat. Clearly, because of its beneficial effects, GLA is an essential fat. While the research with GLA used by itself is impressive, note that for the long term, both essential fatty acid families (Omega-6 and Omega-3) should be used together for optimum health and the good prostaglandin benefits.

Studies now show that the addition of certain fats—from both groups—to the diet assists weight control, cardiovascular disorders, and a host of hair, skin, and nail conditions. Essential-fat deficiencies are linked to a weakened immune system that offers a defenseless home for viral, parasitic, and bacterial invaders that lead to modern day health problems.

The Solution

You can see why the key to my diet is none other than fat. Without it, more food is needed to satisfy your appe-

tite and meet energy needs. Fat in the diet gives a sense
of fullness, or satiety. When the body is fat-starved, one
is hungry all the time, tending to overeat and binge particularly on carbohydrates (cookies, cakes, rolls, bagels,
muffins). Excessive eating of grain carbohydrates (found
in bread, cereal, and pasta, for example) can irritate the
intestines if their intake is much greater than other foods
because of sensitivity to gluten. The popularity of high-
carbohydrate diets has magnified gluten sensitivity.

With small amounts of the correct fats, appetite will
normalize, your weight will stabilize, and you will burn
calories more efficiently. The natural result of all these
efforts is lasting weight loss.

In a similar vein, this book will explain how the role of
cholesterol in the diet and in the bloodstream has been
unduly maligned. An elevated serum cholesterol level is
a signal of improper fat metabolism caused primarily by
too much processed fat. Our bodies need cholesterol for
hormones, nerve impulse transmission, arterial lining,
and bile salts for fat digestion. Did you know that over 80
percent of the brain's solid matter is made up of cholesterol? Just as not all fat is bad, neither is cholesterol all
bad. Cholesterol is such a vital substance to the body that
if sufficient amounts are not ingested from the diet, the
body's own tissue (primarily the liver) will produce more
to compensate for dietary lack. If there is too much absorbed from the diet, then the body will make less.

The unique Fat Flush program (see chapter 17, "The
Two-Week Fat Flush") will remove accumulated and un-
necessary fats and unhealthy cholesterol buildup from
your system. This two-week program highlights three
major points:

Essential fat (in the form of flaxseed oil and dietary GLA
    supplements)
Fiber (contained in raw vegetables)
Fluid (10 glasses of water daily) This will prepare your
    body for the long-term MASTER MENU PLAN.

Each of these components has unique fat-fighting
properties. For example, Long Life Cocktail, (see p. 174)

with its cranberry juice base that acts as a carrier for powdered psyllium husks, is a powerful solvent that simultaneously dissolves unwanted fatty globules in the bloodstream and tissues and delivers beneficial fiber.

THE MASTER MENU PLAN goes beyond the *art* of cooking and explains the *science* of cooking. The 21-day sample menu plan (see "21-Day Master Menu Plan," p. 182) is just that—a sample plan to give you an idea of how to put together a safe and healthy diet. The MASTER FORMULA preceding the plan can be used as a reference for your own menu planning and food selection. For this purpose, as well as to assist professionals in therapeutic diet planning, I have included an exchange list at the end of this recipe section ("Food Equivalents," p. 224). In addition to providing a 21-day sample menu plan and recipes, there is emphasis on the purchase, preparation, and storage of foods. These areas have a major impact on the quality of essential fat. Proper purchase, preparation, and storage will ensure the essential fat value of your diet and weight loss maintenance.

And what about exercise? The exercise plan represents another progression beyond most other exercise programs in that the *Beyond Pritikin* Exercise Plan (chapter 13) is based first and foremost around sunlight. The aerobic exercise of choice is brisk walking. It is most desirable to do your walking outdoors in daylight, if possible, for at least 30 minutes a day. As long as it is done outdoors for a vigorous half-hour at least three times a week, you are following the basic exercise requirement. The outdoors is important here because of the added benefit of full-spectrum light of the sun directly reaching the retina of the eye. When sun strikes the retina, a valuable electrical impulse is carried through the optic nerve to the mental, emotional, and physical centers of the brain. The physical center directly stimulates the temperature-regulating hypothalamus gland, which in turn stimulates the pituitary and pineal glands, which control all other endocrine functions. So, do not wear sunglasses. On the *Beyond Pritikin* Diet, natural sunlight is an important nutrient.

And of course we all know that aerobic exercise is a potent fat burner. The muscle that exercise builds is more metabolically active than fat tissue. While you are exercising, the body releases fat to fuel the muscles. Luckily, this process doesn't end when you stop exercising. Metabolism is raised for several hours after you stop working out.

Several years ago a Pritikin participant sent this poem to me in the mail:

> Lord, grant me the strength that I may not fall
> Into the clutches of cholesterol.
> At polyunsaturates I'll never mutter,
> For the road to hell is paved with butter.
> And cake is cursed and cream is awful
> And Satan is hiding in every waffle.
> Beelzebub is a chocolate drop
> And Lucifer is a lollypop
> Teach me the evils of hollandaise
> Of pasta and gobs of mayonnaise,
> And crisp fried chicken from the South—
> Lord, if you love me, shut my mouth!
>
> (Author unknown)

The *Beyond Pritikin* Diet philosophy, unlike the stringent Pritikin principles, is not about denial. Rather, the *Beyond Pritikin* Diet is a lifelong plan tailored to the lifestyles and nutritional needs of America today. Fat is not to be feared; instead, it's to be better understood. The *Beyond Pritikin* Diet has adapted the basic Pritikin concepts to the latest research on the essential dietary role of fat for better health. The original Pritikin principles that have revolutionized our eating habits in the past decades have now been expanded to ensure a healthy future of easier weight loss, continuous weight maintenance, and a fortified immune system.

4

ALL ABOUT ESSENTIAL FATS

Life is largely a matter of chemistry.
—WILLIAM J. MAYO, M.D.

In order to identify the essential fats among all other fats, we need to understand more about fats in general and answer two important questions:

1. How have fats been optimally designed to work in the body?

2. How can fats become destructive rather than constructive dietetic elements when damaged by food processing and cooking?

Damaged fats are unnatural substances that are biochemically inactive and cannot be utilized by the body. They interfere with the metabolism of natural fats and thereby impede every function of the human body, right down to the cellular level. They weaken cell membranes, suppress the immune system, and block the prostaglandins that act as the "master switch" that regulates and controls almost all cellular activity second-by-second.

Ironically, the smallest changes in the molecular structure of natural fats can have devastating effects on body chemistry. As you will learn, as I did, this can mean the difference between effortless weight loss or weight gain, regeneration or degeneration, health or disease. These differences, and what distinguishes good fat from bad, are what essential fat is all about.

The most direct way to learn about essential fat is to start with some fundamental concepts and simple biochemistry. So, let us begin with the basic definition that all fats, essential fats included, are known as *lipids*. Lipids include fats, oils, and fatlike substances that are greasy, such as cholesterol, butterfat, and vegetable oil, for example. Lipids are not water soluble, but are soluble in alcohol, detergents, and organic solvents like gasoline.

When we speak of fats, we refer to both fats and oils. The difference between them is that fats are solid at room temperature, whereas oils are liquid. Dietary fat is available primarily from two basic sources: animal and vegetable. Animal fats tend to be solid and vegetable fats tend to be liquid.

Fats, proteins, and carbohydrates are the three fundamental building blocks for creating and maintaining life. Each of these three nutrient groups contains the basic chemical elements of life itself: hydrogen, carbon, and oxygen. Compared with protein and carbohydrates, fats contain less oxygen and more available carbon and hydrogen. Since carbon and hydrogen can be burned for energy, fats are our most concentrated energy source and have more calories per gram. Fats contain 9 calories per gram, as compared with 4 calories per gram from proteins and carbohydrates. A little fat goes a long way and has greater staying power than the other nutrient groups. It is ideally used with some protein and complex carbohydrates.

Basic Fat Groups

There are three primary fatty acid types: saturates, monounsaturates, and polyunsaturates. All foods contain a mixture of all types of fatty acids, but one usually predominates. The predominant fatty acid determines how fats are classified.

Here are the fats:

Saturates	Animal sources: pork, lamb, and beef fats (lard, tallow, suet) organ meats, full-fat dairy products such as whole milk, cream cheese, ice cream, and butter. Vegetable sources: coconut oil, cocoa butter, palm oil, and palm-kernel oil, found in commercially prepared baked goods, pie fillings, nondairy cream substitutes, and fast-food preparation.
Monounsaturates	Vegetable, legume, and seed sources: olive oil, avocado, peanut, and canola oil. (Canola oil is similar to rapeseed oil, the most popular cooking oil in eastern Europe, China, India, and Canada.)
Polyunsaturates (Omega-3)	Animal sources: mother's milk, marine oils from salmon, mackerel, herring, cod, sardines, rainbow trout, shrimp, oysters, halibut, tuna, sablefish, bass, flounder, and anchovies; cold-water fish such as trout and crappie. Vegetable sources: flaxseeds, hemp seeds, soybeans, walnuts, wheat germ, wheat sprouts, fresh sea vegetation, leafy greens.
Polyunsaturates (Omega-6)	Animal sources: mother's milk, organ meats, lean meats. Vegetable sources: safflower, sunflower, corn, soy, cottonseed, ses-

ame, raw nuts and seeds, legumes, spirulina, leafy greens.
Botanicals: borage, evening primrose, black currant seeds, and
gooseberry oils.

How Fats Work in the Body

At their biochemical best and in nature's form, fats serve
many invaluable functions. They are the most potent energy source available to the body. Gram for gram, fat
yields more than twice as much energy as either carbohydrate or protein. *As storage for the body's excess calories, all excess carbohydrate and protein calories are also
stored as body fat.*

Fats are the major constituent of all cell membranes
in the body. By maintaining strong cell membranes, they
help protect against invading allergens, bacteria, and viruses. The cell membranes are the body's defense system. Increased permeability can have devastating effects
on any body tissue, allowing toxins a passageway into the
bloodstream.

In babies, fat is needed in the formation of myelin—a
specialized membrane that protects the nerves and is
essential to the normal development of the central nervous system and the brain. This development is best met
by the fat contained in breast milk. Second best is the fat
derived from vegetable oil added in formula preparation. The use of skim milk in the diet of a child younger
than age 2 is not recommended because of the need for
essential fatty acids. At all other ages human beings must
get essential fats through certain unprocessed vegetable
oils, nuts, seeds, and fish sources.

Perhaps the most important role of fats is in the manufacture of prostaglandins (see chapter 6, "The *Beyond
Pritikin* Diet Prostaglandin Protection"), hormonelike
compounds that regulate every function in the human
body at the molecular level. Because the system does not

store prostaglandins, each cell needs a daily amount of essential fat to produce them.

Besides the powerful prostaglandin production, there are other life-supporting functions of fat. These include:

- Assisting the body in utilizing the B vitamins for digestion, nerve health, energy, and mental well-being

- Elevating calcium levels in the bloodstream and transporting it to the tissues for strong bones and cramp-free muscles that are toned and firm

- Carrying and storing fat-soluble vitamins such as A, D, E, and K for healthy skin, reproduction, and blood clotting

- Activating the flow of bile (a fat digestant in the gall bladder)

- Helping the body conserve protein to rebuild vital tissues

- Assisting in maintaining normal temperature

- Insulating and cushioning the vital organs, nerves, and muscles against shock, heat, and cold

- Sealing in moisture for healthier skin, hair, and nails

- Slowing down the absorption of carbohydrates, thus providing more balanced blood sugar levels.

In terms of cooking, fat is an irreplaceable assistant. Salad dressings, stir sautés, and marinades taste flat without the rich flavor that fat imparts. Fat is one of the most vital ingredients in a health-conscious kitchen because it seals in delicate food flavors, keeps food hot, and contributes to juiciness, color, and texture.

Happily for all of us, a diet with healthy fats leaves you satisfied. Fat delays hunger by depressing gastric secretion and slowing down the emptying time for the stomach. Because fats are more slowly digested, they leave you satisfied longer. You don't have to use willpower to push away that sugary desert—you'll be too full!

The Infamous Four

The question is: Why aren't all fats considered healthy fats? The answer can be found in the commercial oil-processing plant and in the privacy of your kitchen.

A fat can be damaged by four invisible factors that I call the Infamous Four: (1) heat, (2) hydrogenation, (3) oxygen, and (4) homogenization. Unfortunately, we often cannot see, taste, or smell the damage caused by these factors, yet all of them create unnatural changes in fatty acid structure. It is important to recognize these four factors so you can protect your foods from them by proper selection, preparation, cooking, and storage practices. Avoiding damaged fats will assist you in optimizing weight loss, beauty, and immunity, as well as protecting you from degenerative disease.

The Heat Factor

Oils are commercially processed to improve shelf life, flavor, smell, and color. They are purified to remove the fat-soluble agricultural residues so prevalent in major food crops such as soybeans, wheat, and corn. Unfortunately, due to the high temperatures involved (sometimes up to 475 degrees), polyunsaturated fatty acids are converted from the naturally occurring, beneficial "cis" form to the unnatural, harmful "trans" form. Cis fats melt at 55 degrees, below the body temperature of 98.6, which makes them fully available to the system. Trans fats, on the other hand, melt at up to 111 degrees, so they remain solid, and therefore unmetabolized, in the human body.

The Hydrogenation Factor

The hydrogenation process that converts liquid oils into hardened fats, such as margarine and vegetable shortening, destroys natural fatty acids in even greater numbers by converting the natural fatty acid form into the biologically impaired trans form. While hydrogenated oil may be more stable than unhydrogenated oil, the trans-fat factor strips the essential fatty acids of their biological potency. Trans-fatty acids cannot be used by the body to produce prostaglandins and furthermore impair the normal use of cis-fatty acids. Trans-fatty acids are rarely found in nature but are predominant in commercial salad oil (15 percent) and hydrogenated products such as margarine (30 percent) and shortening (47 percent). French fries contain about 40 percent trans fats (about the same as doughnuts) while commercial cookies and crackers can range from 30 to 50 percent.

The Oxygen Factor

Oils are more susceptible to oxygen once they have been extracted from their source. Interaction with oxygen creates peroxides, or free radicals, that cause rancidity. Oxygen then becomes less available for its major bodily roles of respiration and detoxification.

Unsaturates are more sensitive to oxygen than saturates due to their biochemical composition of double bonds. ''Poly'' unsaturates contain multiple double bonds and therefore have more potential sites to which oxygen can attach. They are more likely to become oxidized or rancid than either the saturates or monounsaturates. In other words, the more unsaturated an oil is, the quicker it can become rancid.

The oxidation of oils also is related to temperature. Refrigerated oils do not become rancid as quickly as when they are left out at room temperature. Heated oils oxidize very rapidly. At frying temperatures (above 300 degrees), polyunsaturated oils not only rapidly oxidize but are converted from the cis form to the "trans" form. The commercial practice of reusing frying oils raises the specter of both trans and oxidized fats to the most dangerous levels.

Exposure to air when using or storing oil is another way for oxygen to enter the scene. Natural oils contain substances called antioxidants that protect the oil from rancidity; however, these substances, like lecithin and vitamin E, are removed or destroyed during the refining process.

Polyunsaturates can also oxidize inside the body. They can react with normal byproducts of cellular metabolism as well as environmental pollutants such as smog, X rays, cigarette smoke, chemicals, exhaust, and trace metals such as copper, nickel, and iron.

Technically, when polyunsaturates oxidize, they produce "free radicals," a term that has become synonymous with cell and tissue destruction. Free radicals are actually highly reactive molecular fragments that are in search of stability. They need electrons for their stability, and they try to pick them up from other molecules, creating a chain reaction that damages the cells. Normal cells take on a burnt appearance. Premature aging, heart disease, cancer, and other degenerative processes are the result of unbridled free radical activity.

This free radical degeneration will continue unless the free radicals are neutralized by antioxidant substances that pair up their electrons. These substances are vitamins E and C, beta carotene, selenium, and the body's own enzymes.

The Homogenization Factor

Homogenization, a process that extends shelf life, is another common technique that damages fats. Normal milk fat occurs in large globules that are usually digested intact in the intestinal tract. Homogenization breaks up these fat globules into extremely small droplets (one-third the original size) that are dispersed into the milk.

According to leading cardiac specialist and researcher, Dr. Kurt A. Oster, Chief of Cardiology Emeritus at Park City Hospital, Bridgeport, Connecticut, much of the homogenized fat particles can bypass digestion and absorb directly into the bloodstream, carrying with them a destructive enzyme called xanthine oxidase (XO), that is protected by liposomes (membranelike packets). As it is carried through the bloodstream, XO can damage the arteries by attacking plasmalogen, an integral part of the artery wall and heart disease. This results in a lesion on the artery wall. The weakened tissue then attracts cholesterol and fat, which coat the arterial lesion, soothing and smoothing the injury to promote healing. When this happens, plaque buildup results and coronary disease occurs because of constriction created by the concentration of cholesterol. Cholesterol can be compared to the Good Samaritan at the scene of the crime.

The primary opposition to Dr. Oster's XO theory comes from researchers who argue that the XO molecule is simply too large to be absorbed into the bloodstream without first being destroyed by the digestive process. Dr. Oster counters with the fact that the fatal food-poisoning bacteria that causes botulism is even larger than XO and yet is somehow absorbed into the bloodstream without first being destroyed in the digestive tract.

Besides xanthine oxidase, there are other reasons for avoiding milk. Milk may be a contributing cause of arthritis, allergy, and asthma. It may be helpful to eliminate all dairy products for at least three weeks if you have any of these problems. If your condition improves, then look for milk substitutes for a longer time.

Many people are concerned about osteoporosis and so drink milk for its high calcium content. It is interesting to note, however, that those countries that have the highest consumption of dairy products—the United States, Finland, Britain, Sweden, and Israel—also evidence the highest rates of osteoporosis. There are other minerals besides calcium that may be just as important in the prevention and management of osteoporosis. Manganese is one of them.

Dr. Paul Saltman, at the University of California at San Diego, evaluated blood and bone samples of women with severe osteoporosis and women with no sign of osteoporosis. The only striking difference was the blood levels of manganese in the two groups. The osteoporotic women had a manganese level one-quarter of the level of the other group. Manganese deficiency has also been linked with diabetes because of its connection with insulin release. Besides blood sugar, manganese deficiency is connected to disk problems and cartilage formation. Manganese can be found in red meat, nuts, seeds, eggs, and salad greens.

On the *Beyond Pritikin* Diet only nonfat milk (skim milk) that reads 0 fat grams on the label is recommended. Without any fat, there is no XO that can be carried into the body's tissues. Low-fat milk (the 2 percent variety), with a 5-gram fat content per cup, actually derives 36 percent of its calories from fat and thus contains a sufficient fat content to be a potent XO carrier. If you insist on continuing to drink 2 percent milk, boil it before drinking. Heat deactivates XO.

5

THE *BEYOND PRITIKIN* DIET WEIGHT LOSS CONNECTION

The popularity of dieting proves that people will go to great lengths to avoid going to great widths.
—CARL OTTAVI
newspaper columnist and humorist

Yes, obesity is increasing, as I discussed in the expanded Introduction: obesity, a major national health problem, may be easily overcome with essential fats without the health risks associated with dieting. Despite the myriad diets and the abundance of fitness information, America has been growing even fatter. Look at the facts:

• Ninety percent of all Americans think they are overweight.

• Ninety-seven percent of people who go on a diet regain all the weight or more within two years.

• Approximately 15 percent of children and 20 percent of teens are overweight.

• About 25 percent of men and women between the ages of 20 and 74 are clinically obese (i.e., 20 percent above normal weight).

• Over 35 percent of dieters have a goal of losing 15 pounds or more.

Although fewer people now confess that they are actually dieting, Americans are still preoccupied with losing weight. Unfortunately, going on a fad diet usually creates what is referred to as the yo-yo syndrome, whereby the dieter later regains more weight than was originally lost. The cycle of sizable weight loss/gain results in higher and higher weight regain. During the weight loss phase of crash diets, both muscle tissue and fat are lost. During the rebound phase, the weight regained is pure fat. This results in an increase in the size of fat cells and a greater capacity for storing fat.

When calories are abruptly restricted, there is another negative consequence: the body slows down its metabolic rate to allow it to function on less energy, and therefore fewer calories are burned. This process was evolved in our ancestors to allow them to survive the long famines that were common in those times.

There is recent evidence that every time a dieter loses and regains weight, plaque is deposited in the arteries, which leads to atherosclerosis, a prime underlying cause of heart disease. On severely restricted diets, heart muscle tissue can also be lost, causing irregular heartbeat and other more serious dysfunctions. While quick-weight-loss fad diets have proliferated, the statistics show we are not winning the war on fat.

The problem in America is one of excess. Obesity is rated our Number One health hazard that underlies most of our degenerative diseases. In 1984 the Department of Health and Human Sciences released some statistics about the major causes of death in America. The numbers are as follows: (Do be aware that the percentages add up to more than 100 percent. This is because, oftentimes death is due to multiple causes.)

Causes of Death in the United States

Stroke	76.6%
Heart disease	37.4%
Cancer	22.1%

Accidents	4.5%
Lung disease	3.4%
Pneumonia, influenza	2.9%
Diabetes	1.8%
Suicide	1.4%

Most of these leading causes of death are weight related. The obese are at greater risk to heart and circulatory diseases, cancer, respiratory problems, diabetes, and accidents. Other risks include greater surgical complications and pregnancy difficulties. The more overweight, the greater the risk. Excess fat strains every organ in the body.

For many people, it is extremely difficult to lose weight. When calories are restricted, our metabolic rates can adjust downward, matching the lack of food. As previously mentioned, we inherited this response from our ancestors, who needed to be able to survive seasonal fluctuations in food availability. This mechanism is especially active in women because of the added energy demands of bearing children. Because of this, simply restricting calories is often ineffective for lasting weight loss.

Effective weight loss requires affecting your metabolic rate. In my practice, I found that many women were effortlessly losing weight when taking supplements of an essential fatty acid for premenstrual symptoms such as fluid retention, cramps, and irritability. In some way, this essential fatty acid was stimulating their metabolic rates. In the scientific literature there is a study that shows that evening primrose oil enabled individuals at least 10 percent over their ideal weight to lose weight without dieting. Those individuals who were within 10 percent of their ideal weight did not lose weight, indicating that their metabolisms were already at normal efficiency. The key fat nutrient in the evening primrose oil was GLA. It was activating their brown-fat metabolism, or a thermogenic response, as we now call it in the 1990s.

Brown Fat

As you now know, brown fat is a high-energy type of fat whose sole function is to burn calories for heat rather than depositing them for storage. It is your personal *fat burner.* Although brown fat comprises only 10 percent or less of total body fat, it burns one-fourth of all the calories burned by the other fat tissues combined. Brown fat is brown because it contains numerous mitochondria, little fat-burning factories. The rest of the fat in the body is white because it contains few mitochondria. White fat is the insulating layer on the outside of the body, just under the skin. Brown fat lies deeper, surrounding the organs such as the heart, kidneys, and adrenals, as well as the neck, spine, and major thoracic blood vessels. While everybody has a fat burner, they are not all equally active. The thin person who has an actively functioning fat burner can easily convert excess calories into body heat. The obese person, eating the same number of calories, will store them as white fat instead.

In the case of two of my clients, both professional models, it was not until particular salad dressings were added to their diets that those last stubborn 5 pounds were metabolized and lost. For years these women followed the nutritionally chic high-carbohydrate regimens. They ate lots of vegetables, whole-grain cereals, and potatoes without butter. While this routine worked for them in the beginning, after a while their weight reached a plateau and the scale would not budge. They came to me with complaints of dry hair, skin, and nails, and the need to lose more weight for upcoming photo sessions. Within one week of following the *Beyond Pritikin* Diet, the scale finally moved downward. The only dietary change was the addition of two tablespoons of unprocessed safflower oil in the form of salad dressing. Within three weeks, their hair, skin, and nails were noticeably improved. Something remarkable was happening—weight loss and no more hunger pains.

The GLA and the safflower oil that helped weight loss are clearly related to each other. Safflower oil is one of the richest sources of the essential fatty acid cis-linoleic acid. In normal metabolism within the body, cis-linoleic acid is converted into GLA. In many ways, however, this conversion is impaired. If cis-linoleic acid is heated, for example, some of it is converted into trans-linoleic acid, an unnatural fatty acid that not only cannot be converted into GLA but inhibits the conversion of the rest of the cis-linoleic acid into GLA. Safflower oil is frequently heated during commercial manufacturing and in home cooking. Even higher levels of trans-linoleic acid are produced when vegetable oils are hydrogenated into margarines.

Other factors that interfere with GLA synthesis are excessive saturated fats, alcohol, cigarette smoking, caffeine, cholesterol, old age, sugar virus, obesity, diabetes, and deficiencies in zinc, magnesium, vitamins B-6, B-3, C, E, and selenium. These factors are quite common and make the production of GLA from linoleic acid unreliable. This is why preformed GLA is preferred and almost a necessity in this inhibiting day and age.

As a nutritionist, I was taught that we receive plenty of the essential fatty acids—namely, cis-linoleic acid—from dietary vegetable oils like safflower, sunflower, and corn oils. But, as I learned, when oils are processed to extend shelf life or to become margarine, the cis-linoleic acid becomes trans-linoleic acid, a malfunctioning fat. Trans fats are contained in almost all forms of baked products such as breads, cookies, and cakes, where hydrogenated vegetable oil or vegetable shortening appear on the list of ingredients. Without full biological vitality, the refined and altered oils deprive the body of its weight loss capability.

Although the typical American diet is lower in fat calories, at 40 percent, than the original Eskimo diet, at 70 percent, most of our fat comes from damaged fat sources such as commercial vegetable oils (heat damaged), french fries and potato chips (heat damaged and oxidized), margarine and baked goods (hydrogenated), and dairy products (homogenized). None of these food sources is capable of providing fat-burning GLA. These damaged fat sources render fat biologically impotent.

The Big Picture

Fats are everywhere. It is easy to recognize visible fats in foods, but sometimes the fats cannot be identified by sight. While obvious visible fats such as butter, processed vegetable oil, and salad dressing are easier to control, the hidden fats in the creamy cheese sauces, heavily marbled meats, and flaky piecrusts are more challenging to identify. Avoiding the damaged fat that accompanies invisible fat can also be difficult. The best way, of course, to protect yourself from bad fats is to avoid all foods in which the fat source has been heated, hydrogenated, oxidized, or homogenized.

Finding your way through the fat maze therefore takes planning and know-how. To really see more clearly what you're up against, here is a chart that classifies food according to the percentage of calories from fat. Look at the chart to see how much fat is hidden in everyday foods. At this point you need not be overly concerned about being able to identify how much of the hidden fat is also damaged fat. Chapter 18, "The *Beyond Pritikin* Diet Prescription," offers specific guidelines that will keep you on a healthy and essential fat course.

Percentages of Fat Calories Found in Foods

More than 90%	Whipped cream, pork sausage, cooking oils, margarine, butter, gravy, mayonnaise
More than 80%	Spare ribs, bologna, cream cheese, salad dressing

More than 70%	Half and half, peanuts, hot dogs, pork chops, cheddar cheese, sirloin steak, bacon, lamb chops, pecans, macadamia nuts
More than 60%	Potato chips, regular ground beef, ham, eggs
More than 50%	Round steak, pot roast, creamed soups, ice cream, sweet rolls
More than 40%	Whole milk, cake, doughnuts, french fries
More than 30%	Muffins, chicken, cookies, fruit pie, creamed cottage cheese, tuna fish, low-fat milk
More than 20%	Crackers, ice milk, crab meat, beef liver, lean fish
More than 10%	Bread, pretzels
Less than 10%	Sherbet, nonfat milk, most fruits and vegetables, egg whites, baked potato

(Adapted from the Public Health Nutrition Service, Rhode Island Department of Health.)

6

THE *BEYOND PRITIKIN* DIET PROSTAGLANDIN PROTECTION

A salmon a day keeps a coronary away.
—MEDICAL WORLD NEWS

In addition to weight control, the power of essential fats is found in their conversion into prostaglandins. Prostaglandins are short-lived hormonelike substances that regulate metabolic processes throughout the body at the cellular level. They were discovered over fifty years ago in the prostate gland, hence the name prostaglandins. Then, in the 1960s, it was discovered that they were to be found in almost every cell of the body.

The discovery of prostaglandins may be the greatest nutritional finding of the century because of their far-reaching implications. They have been found to control a wide range of activities including immune response, inflammation, reproduction, blood clotting, blood pressure, tumor growth, brain function, and allergies. New properties of prostaglandins are being reported continually. So important and monumental is the prostaglandin connection to health that the 1982 Nobel Prize in medicine was awarded to scientists in prostaglandin research.

Prostaglandins can only be made from two fatty acids: GLA, the Omega-6 fatty acid, and EPA, the Omega-3 fatty acid. These two are the direct prostaglandin building blocks. The prostaglandins formed by GLA and EPA have different functions. Together, the two nutrients form an unbeatable health combination and should be taken together in an approximate ratio of 2:1 (GLA:EPA) for maintenance purposes. However, since nearly 80 percent of all Americans are Omega-3 deficient, it may be prudent to use a 2:1 ratio in favor of EPA for six months to a year to build up body reserves.

Unrefined vegetable oils contain the GLA raw material, cis-linoleic acid, which the body converts to useful GLA. GLA, in turn, produces prostaglandin E1 (known as PGE1) and, to a lesser degree, PGE2 (see The Prostaglandin Factor diagram, p. 54). GLA is directly contained in a few major sources, such as mother's milk, borage, seeds of the evening primrose, gooseberry, and spirulina, a type of plankton.

The direct form of EPA is found in high amounts in cold-water-fish oils from fatty fish such as sardines, salmon, and mackerel. The indirect form of EPA is contained most predominately in the alpha-linoleic-rich flaxseeds. Both forms can convert into PGE3.

Neither the unprocessed vegetable oils nor the Omega-3 fish oils can be converted into prostaglandins without the presence of specific catalysts. Known as enzymatic cofactors, these catalysts are vitamins B-3 (niacin), B-6, and C, and the minerals magnesium and zinc. Unfortunately, in the typical American diet, deficiencies of these nutrients are quite common because of soil depletion, food processing, and poor eating practices.

The presence of the trans-fatty acids from commercially processed oils, hydrogenated margarines, and fried foods interferes with the transformation of GLA and EPA into prostaglandins. *Without the ability to transform into prostaglandins, the essential fatty acids are biologically worthless.*

There are several other factors that hamper prostaglandin production by blocking the enzyme that transforms cis-linoleic acid into GLA. These factors include saturated fats, cholesterol, aging, alcohol, high blood sugar (diabetes), viral infection, radiation, and aspirin. The following diagram gives a detailed illustration of what substances act as blocking factors to the effective metabolism of prostaglandins from essential fatty acids.

The Prostaglandin Factor

Metabolic conversion of essential fatty acids to prostaglandins and common blocking factors of GLA and EPA production:

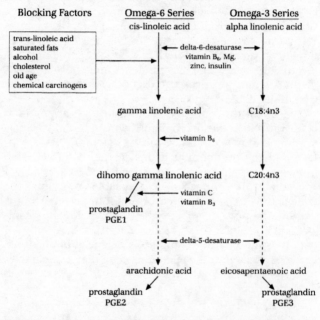

Vitamin Research Products Notes, April 1986, vol. 1, no. 2, 2044 Old Middlefield Way, Mountain View, CA 94043. (800) 541-1623

The Benefits of Prostaglandins

Reports about new uses of essential fats appear almost daily around the world regarding health benefits of prostaglandins. Prostaglandins have single-handedly turned around medicine's negative regard for fat into an extraordinary appreciation of its true biological function. Essential fats may be the savior of twentieth-century disease conditions and immune disorders.

The benefits of essential fats are far-reaching. Reduced cardiovascular disease—America's Number One Killer—has been shown to be related to good fat intake. Fish oils containing EPA are known, for example, to reduce the stickiness of platelets, thereby lowering the chances of unwanted blood clots, the immediate cause of heart attacks and strokes. PGE3 relaxes the blood vessels, preventing arterial spasms and lowering blood pressure. This may also be the mechanism by which migraines are relieved. Fish oils also lower blood cholesterol and triglyceride levels. Populations such as the Eskimos and coastal Japanese consistently eat cold water fatty fish and subsequently have a much lower incidence of all forms of cardiovascular disease.

The high blood sugar associated with diabetes results in high triglyceride (fat) levels in the blood. EPA and PGE3 lower triglyceride levels, thereby decreasing the incidence of vascular disease affecting the hearts, kidneys, and eyes of diabetics. Since insulin deficiency is a common blocking factor of both GLA and EPA formation, supplementation may prove to be a blessing to diabetics who suffer from deficient prostaglandin functioning characterized by nerve twitching, infection, and sexual dysfunction.

Researchers are now studying the Omega-3 fish oils in the prevention and treatment of cancer. The therapeutic activity of beneficial prostaglandins may protect against cancer by strengthening the immune system.

It is important to point out, however, that not all prostaglandins are good. While some suppress inflammation, others actually stimulate it. The prostaglandin known as PGE2 causes inflammation and is produced from arachidonic acid (see diagram, p. 54), a common fatty acid found in land animal meats, liver, and egg yolks. PGE1 and PGE3, on the other hand, produced from unrefined vegetable oils, flaxseed oil, and marine fish oils, suppress inflammation. It is obvious that because the inflammatory prostaglandins are synthesized from different essential fatty acids contained in various foods, diet affects prostaglandin production and the level of inflammation. Excessive red meat and organ meats have the potential of creating the inflammatory type of prostaglandins. Since many diseases have inflammation as an underlying condition, it is important to restrict the intake of these foods.

Early essential fatty acid studies involving linoleic acid showed marginal improvements in cases of eczema, psoriasis, and acne. Recent work with GLA and EPA have shown much better results, especially in combination with zinc and vitamin A. Bottle-fed babies with eczema respond very rapidly to oral and topical application of GLA-containing oils. One multiple sclerosis patient with eczema showed great improvement on GLA. The eczema returned when GLA was discontinued, and again disappeared when GLA was resumed. My patients frequently report that they receive compliments on their complexions when they follow the *Beyond Pritikin* Diet, which promotes essential-fat intake. Their nails are also strengthened and dandruff flaking disappears.

The good news continues. Arthritics experience less pain and joint stiffness when consuming fish oils. Both GLA and EPA seem to significantly slow the progression of multiple sclerosis, an inflammatory autoimmune disease of the central nervous system.

By incorporating into the structure of the cellular membrane, essential fats decrease the permeability of vital tissues and organs. In the case of systemic yeast infection, this is particularly helpful. Essential fats can prevent yeast from spreading into the bloodstream from its normal intestinal and/or vaginal environs. The yeast cannot pass through the intestinal walls into the circulatory system when the mucous membrane lining of the digestive tract is strengthened by essential fats.

Omega-3 and Omega-6 fatty acids are also centrally involved in numerous brain disorders including schizophrenia, depression, and hyperactivity. Essential fat supplementation can reduce alcohol withdrawal symptoms and lessen the severity of hangovers.

A word to the wise is in order here. Although studies often feature the Omega-6s alone or the Omega-3s alone, it is biochemically best to take them together. GLA, taken by itself over time, can result in arachidonic acid production and then the accompanying bad prostaglandin. Conversely, too much fish oil alone can inhibit blood clotting and make you bleed continuously. Exclusive intake of flaxseed oil can result in Omega-6 deficiency after about two years. Moderation is a good nutritional watchword always to keep in mind.

So many diseases are being linked to essential fat metabolism and the prostaglandins every day that this discussion will no doubt be incomplete by the time you read this book. As an example, it was recently found that dry eyes and mouth responded to GLA supplementation. The normalization of tear production is certainly good news for contact lens wearers whose eyes are chronically dry and irritated.

However, a challenge remains: to translate the new clinical findings from laboratories all over the world into practical dietary guidelines that the American public can understand and follow. I think the essential fatty acids should be incorporated into salad dressings, pizza, and even ice cream. Well, the *Beyond Pritikin* Diet is at least a first step in that direction.

7

POLYUNSATURATES: GOOD FATS GONE BAD

Nutriment is not nutriment if it have not its power . . .
Nutriment in name, not in deed.
—HIPPOCRATES

Commercially processed vegetable oils have suffered the same nutritionally deprived fate as processed whole-grain products. A pamphlet entitled "The Oil Story" from the Organic Merchants Association points this out quite graphically:

> The process of refining oils is exactly analogous to the refining of whole wheat, and whole sugar, into white ones. In all cases, one takes a product full of natural vitamins, minerals, enzymes and other food factors, and reduces the original natural food into a relative non-food, devitalized and stripped.

Despite their poor nutritional status, the consumption of vegetable oils has increased dramatically in recent years. In 1960, Americans consumed an average of forty-five pounds of oils per year per person. By 1980 the figure had jumped to sixty pounds. In 1978 there were over three hundred brands of vegetable oil on the market. This increase has been due largely to oil company advertising campaigns that hype the cholesterol-free state of vegetable oils. Vegetable oils are naturally cholesterol-free because cholesterol is found only in animal foods, not vegetables.

Oils were not always as nutritionally deprived as they are today. In the early 1900s, vegetable oils were made by pressing seeds, beans, and vegetables with large rollers. This cold-pressed oil was a healthy, whole substance rich in nutrients from the original food sources, high in lecithin, magnesium, and vitamins E and B-6. This nutritious oil had several economic drawbacks, however. First, the pressing method left too much oil in the pulp. Next, the oil itself became rancid quickly and needed refrigeration for storage. Last, it was strongly flavored, dark in color, and cloudy with sediment. So, in the 1920s, more complex refining procedures were introduced involving heating practices and chemical solvents that increased oil yield, improved stability, lightened color, and removed odor. This made for increased consumer appeal and better marketability. The more highly refined oils did not become rancid and so gained a longer shelf life. They required no refrigeration and so could be transported all over the country without freshness problems. The tasteless, colorless, aroma-free oil was more attractive to consumers who equated uniformity in color, taste, and texture with product wholesomeness. Consumers made the same mistake in choosing white flour over whole-wheat flour.

The health drawbacks of these modern processing methods were subtle but far-reaching. They removed nutrients and added unhealthy trans fats and solvent residues to a once healthy food.

Because of the higher heat generated, the beneficial cis form of essential fatty acids was converted into the unnatural trans form. Remember, trans fats prevent linoleic acid from activating into the GLA so vital for weight loss and the prostaglandins that control every cell in the body.

Even oils inaccurately labeled "cold pressed" have been extracted by the expeller or mechanical method that exposes the oil to temperatures ranging from 140 to 160 degrees. Furthermore, high temperatures are also used to precook seeds and break down tough outer layers for better oil yield. The term *cold pressed* is misleading to some degree because heat is involved in the cooking and pressing process, but it does mean that the oils have not been exposed to chemical solvents.

Most of the vegetable oils found on supermarket shelves are extracted with chemical solvents such as hexane, a chemical relative to gasoline. Hexane has irritating effects on the central nervous system and the lungs.

Both the expeller-pressed and solvent-extracted oils must go through further stages of purification to make them safe for human consumption. They are degummed to remove free fatty acids, then bleached and deodorized to remove pesticides and herbicides containing lead and arsenic, which are fat-soluble.

To ensure the most suitable oil for dietary use, look for the words *expeller pressed* or *crude* on the label. Remember that "crude" *does* mean purified of environmental contaminants. These words signal that the basic oil at least has not been solvent-extracted.

Keep in mind that commercial mayonnaise is made from heat-damaged, processed oils, as are corn chips, potato chips, and liquid egg substitutes. Numerous other condiments, such as tartar sauce, horseradish sauce, salad dressing, mayonnaise substitutes, and low-calorie mayonnaise usually contain processed oils. Furthermore, partially hydrogenated or hardened vegetable oils can be found in all margarines and most cookies, crackers, pie crusts, taco shells, dips, dessert toppings, cocoa and coffee mixes that use water instead of milk, nondairy coffee creamers, candy bars, and some frozen vegetables with sauce and some other frozen food entrees.

What Are the Essential Fats?

Essential fats are polyunsaturates that are properly manufactured to retain whole-food values. They are unhydrogenated and stored without exposure to heat or oxygen. Because polyunsaturates are more susceptible to heat, oxygen, and light due to the greater number of double bonds, they should be consumed raw or in no-heat recipes and should not be used for cooking, and especially not for frying.

The daily amount of essential fatty acids recommended for optimum health for most people can be found in about two tablespoons of essential fat. The obese, children, pregnant women, and those recovering from burns or surgery require more essential fatty acids. For those who want to get their EFAs from food, I suggest a tablespoon of flax and a tablespoon of safflower oil daily. Some people swear by one tablespoon of flax and four evening primrose capsules daily. Remember that a 2:1 ratio is ultimately recommended in favor of an Omega-6 source for healthy people.

Margarine: From Bad to Worse

Vegetable oils that are hydrogenated are made into margarine and shortening by the addition of hydrogen atoms (see the diagram below). While most vegetable oils are slightly hydrogenated, margarine can be partially or fully hydrogenated. The hydrogenation process gives the product a longer shelf life and raises its melting point. This allows liquid vegetable oils to be turned into solid margarine. Vegetable shortening, the most highly hydrogenated product, lasts forever. Its long shelf life is a phenomenon of unnaturally saturated trans fat.

Hydrogenated fats offer many cooking conveniences at the expense of health, as we soon shall see. Convenience factors resulting from the hydrogenation process include an extended shelf life and neutralization of strong odors, tastes, and flavors. Hydrogenated vegetable shortenings are great for baking, and because of their durability they are very economical for large-scale institutional cooking and baking.

The Hydrogenation of Unsaturated to Saturated Fats

Unsaturated   Saturated

Vegetable shortening was first developed in the early 1900s by the English, who used whale oil in their product. By 1911, hydrogenated cooking fat from cottonseed oil was being sold commercially in the United States by Procter & Gamble under the product name Crisco. The miraculous new process of hydrogenation spawned a whole new industry and way of life in the ensuing decades.

"Butterine," the early name for Oleo margarine, was introduced in the 1930s. At that time, Oleo was a white shortening. Early margarine sales were slow, however, probably because consumers didn't like the lardlike appearance of margarine.

The butter industry fought the coloring of margarine for many years. However, by 1952 colored margarine was legalized in every state except Wisconsin and Minnesota. Later, these two strong dairy states legalized the coloring of margarine and sales boomed.

Today, margarine outsells butter. In its heyday, margarine topped butter sales by 100 million pounds per year. The average American consumes ten pounds of shortening and twenty pounds of margarine per year.

Hydrogenation opened the door to fast food and its deep-fried offerings. Unfortunately, this has opened the door to a new variety of diseases. To begin with, the process of hydrogenation has converted the original naturally unsaturated fatty acids into unnaturally saturated fatty acids and trans fats to a staggering degree, up to 47 percent of some margarines. Trans fats block prostaglandin production. Remember, prostaglandins control vital functions such as blood-fat levels, blood pressure, platelet clumping, and formation of red blood cells.

Perhaps most dangerous of all, these trans fats create weakened cell membranes, which are more permeable to viruses and bacteria of all kinds, seriously compromising the body's defense system. To add insult to injury, trans fats are defective fats that cannot be activated into the prostaglandins, which have such far-reaching metabolic effects throughout the body. Research by Dr. Fred Kummerow confirmed the atherosclerotic effects of margarine on test animals in 1974.

Twenty years later a study by Harvard researchers Walter Willett and Alberto Ascherio found that the trans fats in margarine and in partially hydrogenated oils double the risk of heart attack by lowering the good HDL (which, by the way, saturated fat *does not*) and raising the bad LDL cholesterol. In 1993, Dr. Willett and associates published the results of a study in *Lancet* that tracked almost 90,000 women and found a greater than 50 percent heart disease risk among those who ate high trans-fat foods such as margarine. During that same year, the *American Journal of Cardiology* reported a connection between cardiovascular disease and increased trans-fat levels in the bloodstream.

Now while it's nice to have the backing of Harvard and prestigious journals, researchers like Mary Enig, Ph.D., have been warning us for years about the health hazards of trans fats. Enig implicates the rising cancer rates, including breast and prostate cancer, with the corresponding increase in the consumption of vegetable fat. Furthermore, she states that trans-fat consumption is associated with lower immunity, obesity, increased insulin levels leading to diabetes, and a compromised ability to detoxify drugs and chemicals in the body.

Adding insult to injury, additives such as benzoic acid or sodium benzoate are also added to margarine as antibacterial and antifungal agents. Most suspect of all is the use of nickel in the making of margarine and vegetable shortening. Nickel is a suspected carcinogen and freeradical catalyst.

Finally, some parting words from the Community Nutrition Institute, which reprinted an indictment of margarine and hydrogenation from the "*Entrophy Institute Review*" of Ontario, Canada, in 1980:

> If governments really wanted to do something positive for the arteries of North America, they would ban outright the sale of all products containing trans fatty acids. The margarine, vegetable shortening and salad oil makers for too long have used the cholesterol bogeyman to scare people, all the while slipping them the phony trans acids. . . .
>
> The industry could, in fact, make other molecular misfits for an extra cost of two cents a pound, but they have not bothered, preferring to spend money on advertising the health benefits of their sloppily made polyunsaturates. The sale of these products represents a gross failure, the result of a lack of social responsibility on the part of the industry, a disinterested medical research community, and a compliant government. Such indifference and irresponsibility are not tolerated in Germany, where the population demands and gets trans-free (less than 1%) products.

Today there are "un-margarine" margarines on the market that are completely trans-fat free. Spectrum Spread is made from expeller pressed canola oil and is more spreadable right from the fridge than butter or margarine. Available in health food stores, Spectrum Spread is best used for spreads, low-heat sautéing, and sauces.

If you are still interested in an all-purpose margarine substitute, then why not try butter?

8

THE MONOUNSATURATES AND SATURATES AMONG US

*Don't plant an olive tree if only your grandchildren
are to enjoy it.*
—PEASANT PROVERB

The Monounsaturates

There is good news for food lovers because three of the tastiest cooking oils of all are on the healthy fat list. These are olive, peanut, and avocado oils. Called monounsaturated oils, these oils are more stable at high temperatures and less prone to oxidation than their sister polyunsaturates. The Greeks and Italians have been consuming olive oil for centuries and are known for their low incidence of heart disease.

Produced in California and in countries all over the world, including Portugal, Spain, France, Greece, Italy, Tunisia, and Morocco, olive oil is graded into three categories, which are determined by the method of extraction. These three grades are extra virgin, virgin, and pure. The first two (extra virgin and virgin) can truly be labeled "cold processed" because the hand or hydraulic presses used for extraction generate no heat. Extra virgin, which is the most expensive and ranges from a light green to deep green color, is made with the choicest olives from the first pressing. Virgin oil, similar in color and aroma, is also made from the first pressing but uses a lower-quality olive. Pure olive oil is a combination of refined oils from later pressings.

Research by Dr. Scott M. Grundy, director of the University of Texas Health Sciences Center, has promoted the health value of monounsaturates in the diet. His report in the *New England Journal of Medicine*, March 1986, showed that the monounsaturate type of fatty acid found in olive and peanut oils was more successful at protecting arteries from clogging cholesterol than a low-fat, high-carbohydrate diet. In order to avoid saturated fats—the fat found in butter, cheese, and red meat, for example—people have been turning to carbohydrates, as found in Pritikin-style diets, and/or using polyunsaturated oils from corn and safflower. Now the newly identified healthy fats made from olive and peanut oils give a palatable alternative to the bland, low-fat diets that doctors, dieticians, and nutritionists have been promoting for years.

For health-conscious cooks, the olive and peanut oils produce wonderful culinary results. They make richly satisfying salad dressings and stir sautés. They can also be used in the preparation of baked goods. Peanut oil, because of its milder flavor, is preferred in the making of bread. A word of caution is in order, though. The olive oil is a solid healthy-fat choice because of its long-term track record of healthful use by the peoples of the Mediterranean Basin. Peanut oil does not yet have the same reputation in modern medical circles. Animal tests have shown it to be an artery-clogging substance, and peanuts are high in arachidonic acid, which is connected to inflammatory prostaglandins. It would be wise to emphasize olive oil until peanut oil has been completely exonerated.

Enter Canola Oil

A newcomer to the monounsaturated oils is canola oil sold in supermarkets and health food stores. Canola oil is second only to olive oil in its percentage of monounsaturated fat (62% in canola vs. 77% in olive oil). It is the oil lowest in saturated fat and is a source of the healthy Omega-3's. Derived from rapeseed—a plant seed like the mustard seed—canola is versatile because it is practically flavorless. It is the perfect choice for cutting the full-bodied flavor of olive oil when used half and half. Spectrum Naturals has introduced a Super Canola to the market which has the highest monounsaturated fat (78%) content than any other canola oil and any other oil available today. It is also the lowest oil in saturated fat (6% in Super Canola vs. 14% in olive oil).

The Saturates

While the monounsaturated fats are the current dietary heroes of America, the saturated fats are considered current dietary villains. Called saturated fats because the carbon chains are completely filled with hydrogen atoms, these fats are found in animal foods such as red meats and dairy products, and in vegetable oils such as coconut, palm, and palm kernel. Because they raise serum cholesterol more than do the polyunsaturates, they are considered almost poisonous. Yet, they perform many necessary functions in the body.

Saturated fats are needed for energy storage, to cushion organs against shock, and to insulate vital tissues against the cold. The body's capacity for energy storage in the form of fat cells is an evolutionary marvel. Over millions of years our bodies have adapted to periodic famine by building up an energy reserve. Nature in her wisdom provides extra protection for women for childbearing and nursing by storing extra reserves (fat) in their buttocks and thighs.

And so, the problem with saturated fats is related more to unbalanced consumption as well as cooking techniques than to the fat itself. The two prime sources of saturated fats in our diet come from fast food restaurants and foods that are frozen or processed. Fast foods are a $5 billion a year business. On a typical day, 45 million people are fast feeding. McDonald's alone has sold some 60 billion hamburgers. In the book *Amazing Facts*, I learned that if all those McBurgers were stacked, they would create a pile twenty times the height of the Sears Tower in Chicago, the world's tallest building, which is 1,454 feet tall! The worldwide chain has sold enough milkshakes to fill every gas tank in America!

The French Paradox

Another factor in the saturated fat situation is known as the French Paradox. The French enjoy a diet filled with rich pâtés, cheeses, butter, and cream—foods we are taught to avoid because their saturated fat content can lead to heart disease. Yet the cardiovascular disease death rate in French males is less than half of ours. Some say antioxidant-rich wine is the reason, but a more plausible explanation is the fact that the French ingest much less sugar than we do—around 70 percent less, to be exact. (Americans eat about 133 pounds per person per year.) Too much sugar can be stored as saturated fat in the tissues. So if we take a lesson from the French, fat may not be the bad guy after all.

Fast Foods

Here in America, we not only overindulge in sugar but we also tend to overeat saturated fats because they are separated from their original food source, such as beef tallow, coconut oil, or palm oil, and are used for commercial cooking. Because they are more stable against heat and oxidation than are the polyunsaturates, saturated fats are used in restaurant food production. They become hidden in many deep-fat-fried fast foods such as french fries, onion rings, fish, and chicken. Coconut oil is one of the prime ingredients in fast food shakes and nondairy creamers. It is also one of the latest fats to be victimized by the Center for Science in the Public Interest (CSPI), a Washington, D.C.–based advocacy group. In the spring of 1994, CSPI revealed that most movie popcorn is made in coconut oil—the most saturated fat of all. (See chart.) Jane Heimlich reported in *Health and Healing*, June 1994, that coconut oil, like most natural saturated fats, may not be such a bad thing after all:

> After evaluating the research on coconut oil, I have concluded that this entire popcorn flap is based on such faulty (I'm tempted to say 'phony') information that I can't let it pass without telling you the truth about coconut oil. Here are the facts:

> **The Truth About Coconut Oil**
> * Coconut oil does not raise blood cholesterol. This is a "myth" (to quote George Blackburn, M.D., a Harvard researcher) dating back to early flawed experiments in which animals were fed coconut oil exclusively. The small amount of essential fatty acids that coconut oil lacks was not provided, and consequently the animals' cholesterol levels rose.
>   In more recent experiments in which coconut oil was given as part of a normal mixed-fat diet, animals' cholesterol levels did not increase.
>   "Coconut oil has a neutral effect on blood cholesterol, even in situations where coconut oil is the sole source of fat," said Dr. Blackburn, testifying at a congressional hearing about tropical oils on June 21, 1988.
> * Coconut oil in and of itself does not cause heart disease. Populations that get most of their fat calories from coconut oil, such as the Polynesian Puka puka and Tokelauan islanders, have an exceedingly low rate of heart disease.
>   "These [tropical] oils have been consumed as a substantial part of the diets of many groups for thousands of years with absolutely no evidence of

any harmful effects to the populations consuming them," says Mary G. Enig, Ph.D., an expert on fats and oils who blew the whistle on margarine and other hydrogenated oils.

- Not all saturated fats are bad for you. Coconut oil's saturated fats are made up mostly (65 percent) of medium chain triglycerides (MCTs). (Triglycerides are the chemical forms in which fatty acids occur in vegetable oils.)

  MCTs (also found in palm kernel oil) are easily digested. In fact, patients with malabsorption problems who cannot digest conventional fats are fed Mead Johnson's Portagen, a formula containing MCTs—a fractionated coconut oil. Infant formula containing MCTs is also a lifesaver for premature babies.

- Coconut oil is less likely than other oils to cause obesity because the body easily converts it into energy rather than depositing calories as body fat. You won't get a spare tire around your midsection just from eating foods containing coconut oil.

- Coconut oil kills germs. Like mother's milk, coconut oil contains a component that is antimicrobial. Coconut oil users, who dwell primarily in the tropics, an ideal environment for parasites, are protected from infections. In a recent medical article, Dr. Enig proposed giving coconut and palm kernel oils to AIDS patients.

Why Coconut Oil Is So Maligned

So how did coconut oil become the despised artery-clogging nemesis?

Credit the American Soybean Association (ASA) and its friends. In 1986, the ASA sent a "Fat Fighter Kit" to soybean farmers enjoining them to write to government officials, food companies, etc., protesting the encroachment of "highly saturated tropical fats like palm and coconut oils . . . [which are] not only stealing US soybean markets, but . . . [also] a threat to consumer health."

Center for Science in the Public Interest joined the anti–tropical oil campaign that same year, issuing news releases referring to palm, coconut, and palm kernel oils as "rich in artery-clogging fat."

In October 1988, Nebraska millionaire Phil Sokolof, a recovered heart attack patient and president of the National Heart Saver Association, began running full-page newspaper advertisement accusing food companies of "poisoning America" by using tropical oils with high levels of saturated fat.

Major food companies, sensitive to consumer fear, reformulated hundreds of products, replacing tropical oils with partially hydrogenated oils. Today coconut oil accounts for only 1.0 to 1.3 percent of the U.S. food supply.

If It Isn't Popped in Coconut Oil, Don't Eat It

Next time you go to the movies or a ballpark and want to snack on popcorn, ask the vendor what kind of oil the kernels are popped in. If it isn't coconut oil, it's probably partially hydrogenated vegetable oil, and that isn't good for you.

You can easily make "healthy" popcorn at home using Country Store Popcorn's No. 500 Stovetop Popper Kit (a stovetop popper, popcorn, popcorn salt, and coconut oil cost $38.95), which produces fluffy, tender popcorn in five minutes. Send for a catalog from Wileswood, P.O. Box 328, Huron, OH 44839. Or call (419) 433-3355 or fax (419) 433-7781.

A good source of coconut oil is Omega Nutrition, Bellingham, WA, (800) 661-3529. It offers organic coconut oil, which is ideal for all cooking needs.

If coconut oil has been maligned for economic and political reasons, what other misinformation have you been fed about fats and oils? Plenty!

As it turns out, palm oil, another tropical oil that is falsely maligned, has an even better balance of fatty acids than coconut oil. It is actually a decent source of the monounsaturates (39 percent mono composition, to be exact). The flexibility of both the coconut and palm oils lends them quite nicely to the manufacture of chips and crackers.

Oil or Fat	Percentage of Saturated Fatty Acids
Coconut oil	92
Butterfat	66
Beef tallow	52
Palm oil	51
Lard	41
Cottonseed oil	27

In 1986, McDonald's and Burger King yielded to public pressure by switching from beef fat to vegetable oil for their deep frying. Other chains may follow suit. While their intentions are good, more damaged fats are introduced into the American diet in the form of trans fats. The polyunsaturated vegetable oils that McDonald's and Burger King are using are much more easily damaged at the high frying temperatures (350 degrees). The continuous reuse of the same frying oil results in even more trans fats. The oil goes rancid sooner. The original reason for saturated fats for restaurant use was their stability over polyunsaturates.

The problem with saturated fats is twofold: First, their presence biochemically blocks the essential fatty acid conversion into the beneficial prostaglandins. Prostaglandins have been shown to lower blood cholesterol and triglycerides and to promote overall cardiovascular protection by inhibiting blood clots, dilating blood vessels, and lowering blood pressure. By inhibiting prostaglandins, saturated fats promote heart disease. Second, whenever fat is eaten, bile acids are produced by the liver to aid in fat absorption in the intestines. High-fat diets cause too much bile to be produced. When there is insufficient fiber in the diet, bile acids remain in the digestive system for too long and are changed into noxious substances by bacteria. In America, high-fat diets usually go hand-in-hand with low fiber intake.

Two of the easier solutions to this problem are simply to increase the essential fatty acids and to avoid the fast-food fryer. Another is to eat more fiber. Fiber-rich foods are vegetables, fruits, legumes (peas and beans), and grains (see Chapter 12, "The Lowdown on Fiber").

Convenience Foods

Fast foods are also convenience foods. Frozen dinners and entrees are extremely popular convenience foods. In 1985 there was a 26 percent increase in the sales of frozen dinners and entrees. This was double the 1982 level. According to the same report by Business Trend Analysts, Inc., retail sales of frozen dinners and entrees were thought to reach $4.5 billion in 1986. Convenience foods are increasing in demand because of more people living alone, the increase of working mothers, smaller families, people living longer, and the emphasis on less time spent on food preparation. The microwave oven has spurred sales in frozen foods. In a 1985 poll of seven hundred working women by *Mademoiselle* magazine regarding their shopping and eating habits, it was revealed that while there is an interest and concern about the nutritional quality of food, most are still not making their meals "from scratch." Sixty percent buy frozen foods; 67 percent buy convenience foods; 38 percent eat them three times per week. Recent surveys show that a majority of Americans eat convenience foods at home. According to the *Nutrition Action Health Letter*, a record 42 percent of meals were eaten away from home in 1983, based on a Gallup survey. Based on these statistics, we can see a strong "tendency" toward turning the responsibility of our food selection and preparation over to total strangers.

However, like their restaurant counterparts, frozen food also means hidden fat. *The average frozen food entree contains over 50 percent fat*. We are forced to ask the question, are we eating frozen food or frozen fat?

The chart below details the fat content of frozen dinners and entrees.

Frozen Dinners & Entrees
(Average Over Product Line)

Brand (serving size)	Fat (% of cals)	Calories	Sodium (mg)	Price* (per lb.)	
La Choy Dinners (12 oz.)	10	243	1822	na	
Great Escapes Lite (10 oz.)	15	279	1053	$3.58#	
Light & Elegant (9 oz.)	19	259	880	4.62#	
Benihana (na)	20	347	1311	4.03	LEAN
Armour Classic Lites (11 oz.)	21	265	954	5.10	
Lean Cuisine (10 oz.)	28	260	978	4.11	
Mrs. Paul's Light (10 oz.)	29	254	836	5.80	
Green Giant Entrées (10 oz.)	32	347	996	4.15	
Chun King Dinners (12 oz.)	32	334	na	na	INTERMEDIATE
Legume (11 oz.)	33	265	435	5.17	
Weight Watchers (10 oz.)	35	277	1051	4.93	
Armour Dinner Classics (11 oz.)	39	391	1339	5.16	
Celentano (10 oz.)	40	357	672	4.33	
Swanson 4-Part Dinners (12 oz.)	40	483	1154	2.52	
Patio Dinners (13 oz.)	41	618	na	na	
Hungry man Dinners (17 oz.)	41	728	1772	2.70#	
Hungry Man Entrées (13 oz.)	41	531	1476	na	
Le Menu (11 oz.)	42	398	1001	5.45	
Budget Gourmet (10 oz.)	43	373	849	2.87	FATTY
Swift Internat'l Entrées (6 oz.)	43	358	865	na	
Swanson Entrées (8 oz.)	45	310	908	2.88#	
Banquet American Favorite Dinners (11 oz.)	45	439	1331	1.82#	
Stouffer's Entrées (9 oz.)	46	343	1130	2.56	
Barber Foods (7 oz.)	47	426	957	4.55#	
Banquet Family Entrées (8 oz.)	49	285	989	na	
Old El Paso (na)	55	359	623	4.67	

*Prices obtained in Washington, D.C.
# Average price based on fewer than five items.
na = not available
Source: *Nutrition Action Health Letter*, November 1985.

The conclusion from all this is that fast foods are here to stay. Busy lifestyles simply do not allow much time in the kitchen or supermarket anymore.

Is There a Solution?

Our fat problems are directly related to the effects of contemporary technology on the quality of nutrition, and the resultant effects on health and well-being. While we have the technology to process food and still preserve health, what we have done is to produce food that looks and tastes good, and that is profitable and convenient for the manufacturer, but is unhealthy. As long as the public is willing to buy convenience foods that are high in fat and salt and low in fiber, the manufacturers will continue to make them.

I am pleased to report that I am aware of one food company where food processing has been based on good nutrition for over forty years. The company is Walnut Acres, located in Penn's Creek, Pennsylvania. Walnut Acres is a farm that practices organic farming on five hundred acres of chemical-free soil. They use no pesticides or fungicides in their products. They take special care in the processing of their oils to ensure a fresh, nonrancid, nutritious product. They also have a line of foods that is canned and dried without the use of preservatives or additives. They process their own ingredients on the farm in small batches to ensure freshness. Quality control is complete from start to finish. Walnut Acres is the original direct-from-the-farm natural food provider. Farm-fresh foods are produced daily, and pure, untreated mountain water from deep wells is used in food preparation. It is hoped that the example set by Walnut Acres will serve as a model for large-scale food processing in the future.

9

CHOLESTEROL AND THE *BEYOND PRITIKIN* DIET

There is still some confusion about dietary cholesterol and blood cholesterol. How much cholesterol you eat is not as significant as how much remains in the bloodstream.
—DR. RONALD GOOR,
former official of the National Heart,
Lung and Blood Institute

You might be wondering how cholesterol fits into the *Beyond Pritikin* Diet picture. Well, cholesterol is a friend, not a foe, when treated properly. The real question, then, is how has it been treated? Most important, has it been damaged by heat or oxygen?

Cholesterol is such an important substance that it is contained in practically every cell in the human body and used for many body functions. It helps the body manufacture adrenal hormones and sex hormones in both males and females. It also aids in manufacturing vitamin D and bile acids, which are used for fat digestion. Much of the brain itself is composed of cholesterol, and it also helps form the insulation around nerves. Cholesterol acts as a lubricant to the artery walls to reduce friction in blood flow. In fact, cholesterol is so vital that the liver will produce it on its own if there is not enough entering the body from dietary sources. Almost three-fourths of your cholesterol is made by your liver, whereas one-fourth is derived from the foods in your diet.

Cholesterol is found only in animal fats such as chicken, fish, beef, pork, and lamb, and in animal by-products such as milk, cheese, butter, and eggs. Biologically, no vegetable can contain cholesterol. So, Mazola, Puritan, and other highly promoted vegetable oils aren't proclaiming any unique advantage when they boast that their oil is cholesterol-free. And, while these oils may be truly free of cholesterol, the fact that they are heat treated and refined means they may contain elevated levels of trans fats, which are ineffective in protecting against cardiovascular disease, their advertised role. In fact, these heat-damaged oils may actually hasten cardiovascular disease.

While the oil manufacturers have deactivated the once-beneficial vegetable oils, careless cooking and storage practices in restaurants and on the home front can actually sabotage normally healthful cholesterol foods. According to a 1979 study by Dr. C. B. Taylor in the *American Journal of Nutrition*, oxidized cholesterol from food sources that are left out at room temperature or that are fried, smoked, cured (sausage), or aged (cheese) can be highly atherogenic (plaque producing). It is not pure cholesterol that creates artery-clogging plaque, but rather the toxic substances produced by the oxidation of cholesterol. Oxidized derivatives of cholesterol are unstable and decompose into free radicals, which damage blood vessel walls.

Foods that can cause problems are improperly stored eggs, milk, or butter that are exposed to room temperature for long periods of time and are not stored in tightly sealed containers. Other oxidized cholesterol sources can be found in any fast food fried chicken, fish, and hamburgers. Dried milk, dried eggs, and packaged, dry baking mixes (custards, cakes, puddings, pancakes) are also added to the list. In fact, any animal food that has been exposed to the ravages of oxygen for extended periods of time is likely to contain chemically altered cholesterol. This can be seen in the cooking of eggs. Hard-boiled or fried eggs produce the highest serum cholesterol; scrambled or baked eggs produce less; soft-boiled eggs produce the least.

High-Density Lipoproteins (HDL) and Low-Density Lipoproteins (LDL)

Cholesterol is carried through the bloodstream in two protein fractions, high-density lipoprotein (HDL) and low-density lipoprotein (LDL). The HDL is considered the good cholesterol because it transports cholesterol away from the arterial walls to the liver for disposal, thus blocking its buildup in the blood vessels. The bad cholesterol (LDL) deposits cholesterol in the arterial walls, promoting hardening of the arteries.

It is now highly suspected that the natural metabolic process of oxidation (in which unstable atoms that alter cell membranes are formed, called "free radicals") is what actually makes LDLs harmful. This is why antioxidants such as vitamin E are so important in preventing the atherogenic effect of LDL.

Age	Moderate Risk	High Risk
20–29	greater than 200	greater than 220
30–39	greater than 220	greater than 240
40 +	greater than 240	greater than 260

The ratio between total cholesterol and HDL cholesterol is now considered more important than just the total cholesterol value alone. In addition, there are cholesterol levels which are age-and-sex-dependant that are associated with the increased risk of coronary artery disease. It is interesting to note that women in general have higher average HDL cholesterol levels than do most men (55 mg/dl for women and 45 mg/dl for men). Concurrently, women evidence less coronary heart disease than do males.

A decisive study reported in the *Journal of the American Medical Association* in early 1984, known as the Lipid

Research Clinic's Coronary Primary Prevention Trial, demonstrated that elevated cholesterol levels were connected with heart disease risk factors. This ten-year, $150 million study was the largest, most expensive project in medical history. It concluded that elevated cholesterol levels in the bloodstream were a major risk factor in heart disease. When blood cholesterol levels were lowered, the incidence of fatal heart attacks was reduced. The four thousand men who participated in the study and lowered their blood cholesterol values, either through diet or drugs, lowered their incidence of heart disease and heart attacks. Thus, it is now generally suggested that adult Americans lower their total cholesterol value below 200 mg/dl. The American Heart Association states that most heart attacks occur when blood levels reach between 210 and 265 mg/dl. Children should not exceed 185 mg/dl.

Elevated cholesterol levels are commonly found in liver and cardiovascular disease, diabetes, stress, and low thyroid function. Stress cannot be overlooked as an external factor that can upset body chemistry. The emotional stress factor can also raise cholesterol levels independent of diet. It has also been shown that stress management techniques can lower cholesterol levels, independent of diet. Dr. Meyer Friedman, who conceived the notion of the Type A and Type B behavior system, underscores the stress factor in the development of heart disease. Dr. Dean Ornish echoes agreement in his book *Stress, Diet and Your Heart.*

While much attention has been focused on the danger of too much cholesterol in the bloodstream, the danger of too little has been relatively ignored. Levels far below 180 mg/dl have been correlated with anemia, acute infection, and excess thyroid function. Moreover, significantly depressed cholesterol values have been found in autoimmune disorders. Low cholesterol levels may function as a precursor to impaired immunity, cancer, and higher suicide rates, although this has not been fully substantiated.

Since high blood cholesterol values can be caused by a number of factors such as age, obesity, stress, and cigarette smoking, it is wise to control these factors as much as possible. Losing weight, managing stress, and stopping cigarette smoking are good preventive measures to reduce major risk factors in the prevention of cardiovascular disease.

The ultimate question is, what is the most effective method of lowering cholesterol in the bloodstream? In terms of diet, major researchers believe that it is not dietary cholesterol that raises blood levels, but excessive saturated fats in the form of red meats and whole-milk dairy products. (Plus, don't forget that saturated fats are made by the body itself from excess carbohydrates such as sugar. So too many carbs can create high serum cholesterol as well.) Dr. Michael White, associate director for Prevention, Education and Control at the National Heart, Lung and Blood Institute, states: "Another point of confusion is in thinking that dietary cholesterol is the main culprit. Actually, saturated fats have a greater effect on blood cholesterol." In agreement, Dr. Bruce McManus of the University of Nebraska Medical Center adds that ". . . saturated fat intake above a certain level is as important and probably more important than one's intake of cholesterol in determining your blood levels of cholesterol." These conventional experts essentially agree that it is not the cholesterol itself in foods that creates a high serum level in the bloodstream.

Ever since cholesterol was identified in the 1960s as a component of the fatty deposits found in the inner walls of the arteries, it has been thought that cholesterol was the main culprit in coronary artery disease. However, it was never proved that it was cholesterol that caused the plaque formation in the first place. In the case of cholesterol, association is not necessarily causation. In other words, the presence of cholesterol may be the result of the disease, not necessarily the cause.

Dr. Henry Bieler was the nutritional mentor of actress Gloria Swanson. While she was at the Pritikin Center, she introduced me to Bieler's writings. He defies current convention with his visionary theory about the way in which cholesterol works in the body. In studying Bieler's ideas, I concluded that so much unfavorable publicity has been unjustly directed toward cholesterol that the following passage from Dr. Bieler's book *Food Is Your Best Medicine* is important in clarifying the issue:

During the development of the embryo, cholesterol is supplied by the mother's blood. After birth the child must manufacture its own. The oil needed for this, nature supplies in the most useful fat, cream, otherwise known as butterfat. One of the important functions of the liver is the synthesis of cholesterol from butterfat. Of course, other vegetable and animal fats can be used, but during the child's early development, butterfat is supplied by mother's milk.

The cholesterol, built up by the liver cells from simple fats, circulates in the blood in just the proper concentration to be utilized by the cells which line the artery walls, and is held there as the perfect lubricant. As these cells wear out, they are cast off, together with their cholesterol, and excreted by the body, while new cells grow and absorb new cholesterol from the blood. Thus, there occurs a continuous in-and-out flow of cholesterol, which, as long as the body is in perfect health, is maintained at a specific level.

When the physiological level for the cholesterol is disturbed by a more rapid breaking-down than building-up process, the overall cholesterol concentration in the blood is increased and there occurs a state of *hypercholestremia*, i.e., too much cholesterol in the blood. There are simple laboratory tests by which the amount of circulating cholesterol can be determined.

The only condition that can cause a more rapid breaking-down than building-up of cholesterol is a diseased state of the artery walls. *Overeating of fats and oils, as long as they are in their natural state, cannot cause arterial disease.* The body merely stores the excess as fat.

It is only when "unnatural" fats, or "natural" fats which have been altered by being overheated, are consumed as food that the trouble arises. Especially is the composition of the fat altered when it is heated with starch (for example, French-fried potatoes). I have found that it is impossible for the liver to synthesize a perfect cholesterol from a fat that has been heated with starch. The resulting cholesterol is used by the body for arterial lining, but being an unnatural or altered cholesterol, it fails to wear well, soon breaks down and is corroded, resulting in various forms of arterial disease and degeneration—arteriosclerosis (commonly called hardening or narrowing of the artery walls, which causes them to lose their elasticity); atherosclerosis (fatty deposits on the arterial walls, which may impede or even block the blood flow); coronary thrombosis (blood clotting in the arteries, which blocks the blood supply to the heart); and aneurism (ruptured tumor in the artery wall). In these states the concentration of cholesterol in the blood is much higher than the normal level. The increased level can be detected early by the alert physician as a danger signal which will lead him to make a study of the patient's fat metabolism.*

According to Bieler, elevated serum levels of cholesterol suggest a problem in fat metabolism caused by damaged fats that the body cannot process. Elevated blood levels of cholesterol are not related to a diet high in saturates unless those fats are overheated.

Bieler does not specifically discriminate between heat-damaged saturated fats and polyunsaturated fats. The fact is that polyunsaturates are much more easily damaged by heat and oxidation. Rancid polyunsaturates generate free radicals, which attack the blood vessel walls. The free radicals also stimulate the production of inflammatory prostaglandins. As we've already seen, the

---

*Henry G. Bieler, M.D. *Food Is Your Best Medicine* (New York: Ballantine Books, 1984) pp. 114–115.

trans-fat content of heat-damaged oils suppresses the production of anti-inflammatory prostaglandins, and inflammation becomes chronic. Cholesterol synthesis is increased during inflammation, and it is drawn to the damaged blood vessel walls. The accumulated cholesterol actually protects the damaged blood vessels like a bandage on a wound.

At first it may seem that these different views of fat and health are quite divergent. But they are actually related. It is easy to blame fats in general when it is heat-damaged fats that are the real problem. In the high-fat American diet, higher saturated-fat intake is generally associated with heat-damaged and oxidized fats. Witness the popularity of fast foods and the reuse of frying oils. While studies have linked fat to heart disease, diabetes, and cancer of the breast, colon, and prostate, they have not attempted to determine whether the damage caused by heat, hydrogenation, oxygen, or homogenization is actually responsible.

Likewise, it is easy to blame fats in general when it is heat-damaged polyunsaturates that are the real source of the problem. Because polyunsaturates are more susceptible to oxygen than are saturated fats, they go rancid more quickly. Polyunsaturates are therefore proportionately more responsible for the disease-causing activity of fat. The peroxides formed by rancidity attack cell membranes, enzymes, and DNA. They are responsible for premature aging, skin wrinkling, heart disease, and cancer.

Heat-damaged and hydrogenated polyunsaturates also form trans fats, which have been associated with the same diseases as fats (or heat-damaged fats) have been connected with. Trans fats inhibit beneficial prostaglandin activity and cause chronic inflammation. Trans fats worsen all diseases, accelerating the degenerative processes initiated by rancid fats.

Thus, disease is not the result of cholesterol, saturated fats, or polyunsaturated fats; it's a result of a massive essential fatty acid deficiency that regulates their utilization in the body and the effects of food processing. The destructive effects of heat, hydrogenation, oxygen, and homogenization can affect all of these food constituents. Cholesterol can become oxidized and stale; excessive saturated fats from fast foods and convenience foods can clog the system and block prostaglandin production. Polyunsaturates can become rancid and form free radicals. In these damaged or unbalanced states, these foods cause disease. Unprocessed and taken in moderation, they provide needed nutrition.

Triglycerides

Any discussion of cholesterol would be incomplete without including the triglycerides. Basically the word *triglyceride* can be used interchangeably with *fat* or *oil*. Triglyceride is also the form in which the body stores fat in the connective tissue. That roll above your stomach, for instance, is actually excess triglyceride. In terms of diet, too much refined carbohydrates in the form of white sugar, white flour, and products such as white bread, cakes, cookies, candies, and soda, as well as alcohol, can account for elevation of blood triglyceride levels. Even too much fruit and natural unsweetened fruit juice can elevate triglyceride levels.

Although I am not aware of any clinical studies, I have observed that people who drink more than two cups of coffee per day have difficulty in reducing elevated triglyceride levels. Levels between 70 and 150 mg of triglyceride per deciliter of blood are considered optimally healthy by most nutritionally oriented physicians.

A low triglyceride value, like a low cholesterol value, is not necessarily a sign of better health. When triglyceride values are lower than 70 mg, it may indicate that fatty acids are not being released properly into the bloodstream and there is some low-grade liver dysfunction. Conversely, when triglyceride levels are much greater than 150 mg, it may reflect a diet too high in processed foods or fruits, or a liver problem in which fatty acids are being poorly broken down and utilized in the bloodstream.

High triglyceride values may also be due to thyroid dysfunction, too much alcohol, and medications such as estrogen replacement therapy, diuretics, and beta blockers. Women especially need to be mindful of the fact that high triglycerides are known to increase susceptibility to heart disease—even when cholesterol levels are normal. A low-carbohydrate diet (reduced intake of pasta, potatoes, corn, and rice) plus exercise and weight loss can help lower triglyceride levels.

During my years at the Pritikin Center, I noted that the excessive use of apple juice concentrate as a sweetener to replace all forms of sugar including honey in many of the Center's recipes contributed to high triglyceride levels. Diets that emphasize high amounts of carrot juice or fruits of any kind can induce unusually high triglyceride levels. Excessive sugar in the diet from refined sugar or fruit sources can be stored in the tissues as excess fat.

10

THE *BEYOND PRITIKIN* DIET FOOD CHOICES: WHERE THE ESSENTIAL FATS ARE FOUND

Adequate food is the . . . laboratory of long life.
—DR. CHARLES MAYO

Foods or food supplements that are rich sources of essential fats must be included in the daily diet. The essential fats are required for prostaglandins, which are intimately involved with every cell of the body. Since prostaglandins are destroyed as soon as they perform their duties, a daily supply of essential-fat raw material is necessary to continue the prostaglandin health watch and control. For most people, two tablespoons of essential fat per day is all that is required.

Essential fat is also crucial during the initial weight loss period in order to enable the body to burn calories more efficiently. It is also important after weight is lost to maintain efficient burning of calories.

While unprocessed oils or GLA supplements can help nourish the brown fat I call your fat burner, the Omega-3 rich foods, or EPA supplements, can protect your entire cardiovascular system. They can also increase metabolic rate while ridding the body of excess fluids. In addition to aiding in weight loss and maintaining healthy arteries, eating essential fat foods may alleviate food allergies and depression and strengthen hair and brittle nails.

The GLA Fat Burners

These food sources supply the highest amounts of cis-linoleic acid, which can convert to gamma-linolenic acid in your body:

Unrefined Vegetable Oil	Percentages of Linoleic Acid
Safflower	78
Sunflower	69
Corn	62
Soy	61
Walnut	59
Cottonseed	54
Sesame	43
Rice bran	32
Peanut	31
Olive	15
Coconut	2

Other sources of cis-linoleic acid include green leafy vegetables such as kale, collard greens, and swiss chard, raw nuts and seeds, liver, kidneys, brains, sweetbreads, and lean red meats.

Other direct sources of GLA come from plants. The richest source is borage, at 24 percent GLA. Next is black currant oil at 15 to 19 percent GLA, then gooseberry oil at 10 to 12 percent GLA, and last, evening primrose oil at 2 to 9 percent GLA, depending on the strength of the plant.

Omega-3s

There is a great variety of essential fat available with the EPA Omega-3 food group. Many cold-water fish and seafoods contain sufficiently high amounts of EPA for optimum cardiovascular benefit. The highest concentrations of EPA have been found in north Atlantic sardine oil at 18 percent EPA, while salmon oil contains 9 percent and mackerel oil has about 5 percent. In general, the fatter the fish, the more Omega-3 it contains.

The following chart shows the highest EPA content of selected fish:

Comparison of EPA Content in 3.5 Ounce Servings of Selected Fish

Fish	Milligrams of EPA
Anchovy	747
Salmon, chinook	633
Herring	606
Mackerel	585
Tuna, albacore	337
Halibut, Pacific	194
Cod, Atlantic	93
Trout, rainbow	84
Haddock	72
Swordfish	30
Red snapper	19
Sole	10

The original producers of EPA are the sea vegetation, or plankton, that inhabit Arctic and Antarctic waters. Next in the food chain are krill (shrimplike organisms), which are eaten by the bigger fish. The production of EPA is actually an antifreeze survival mechanism in extremely cold water temperatures. The colder the water, the more EPA is produced. In warmer waters, little EPA is made by plankton.

Besides fresh edible sea vegetation (EPA disappears if the seaweed is dried) and fatty fish itself, land-grown green leafy vegetables are another source. The best source of the EPA precursor alpha-linolenic acid (ALA) is flaxseed. Flaxseed is a star nutrient of the '90s with its

placement as a Designer Food with the National Cancer
Institute. Research is being conducted on the role of
flaxseed in the immune system, for bone mineralization,
and with cholesterol metabolism. Earlier studies by Dr.
Johanna Budwig of Germany confirm flaxseed's role as
a cancer controller and tumor dissolver. Dr. Donald
Budin demonstrated that Omega-3 deficiency is a central
cause of mental illness. Other research has connected
flaxseed's rich Omega-3 content with reversal of problems with growth and motor coordination, tissue inflammation, and arthritis. Here is a comparison of
Omega-3 sources:

Comparison of Omega-3 Sources
Percentage of Alpha Linolenic, Omega-3 by Total
Weight of Seeds

Flaxseed	57%
Chia Seed	30%
Hemp (Sativa) Seed	30%
Pumpkin Seed (East European Seed Type)	15%
Canola Oil	10%
Soybean Oil (Unrefined)	8%
Walnut (Black American)	5%
Fresh Leafy Vegetables (Average Serving)	0.009%

The only natural direct source of both Omega-6 and
Omega-3 is found in mother's milk, whereas cow's milk
is a comparatively low source. When babies were fed
skim milk preparations, their appetites dramatically increased and they consumed twice the amount of formula than infants fed on mother's milk, which is
naturally high in essential fatty acids. When these infants
were put back on a diet of mother's milk, their appetites
normalized.

This indicates that appetite control may be naturally
regulated with the proper dietary fats. For years doctors
have suggested breast-feeding to ensure in children a
strong immune system and freedom from allergies. Now

we know that the EFAs may be the key ingredients in breast milk that are responsible for the healthier breast-fed babies.

For those mothers unable to breast-feed, there is an easy alternative. Essential fatty acids can be absorbed through the skin. You can puncture a GLA capsule, for example, squeeze out the oil quickly to avoid oxidation, and rub it into the baby's abdomen and arms. When the infant is 1 year old and is eating solid foods, the capsule can be opened and mixed with the food.

Essential Fat Dietary Supplements

Encapsulated oils may be the only way for you to include essential fats in your diet if you eat out frequently or eat ready-made frozen foods at home and don't like fish. If these oils are so lacking in the normal diet, then an essential fat in supplement form should be considered a food, not a pill.

Restaurants use either processed heat-treated vegetable oils or hydrogenated vegetable margarines, or both. These substances have no biological value to you and can even thwart GLA utilization in your body. So, while it may be ideal to avoid all of these damaged, unnatural fats, it is really practical to supplement with essential fat to make sure your tissues are properly nourished. It is not enough just to avoid the bad; you still must supplement with the good. When the *Beyond Pritikin* Diet food choices are limited or unavailable, even at home, these supplements offer fat-burning/calorie-processing power.

Caveat Emptor: What the Buyer Should Know About Fish Oil Capsules

Since the fattier fish are the only significant sources of EPA, many individuals will want to supplement their diets with fish oil capsules. What's wrong with eating fresh fish, you say? First of all, people may not want to eat enough of the fatty fish per day to derive the EPA benefits. Second, the higher the fat content in the fish, the more fat-soluble pollutants that can accumulate. This means that the highest EPA-containing fish may also be high in PCBs (polychlorinated biphenyls) and heavy metals such as mercury and arsenic.

If you choose to go the fish oil capsule route, there are several ways to assess the purity and freshness of the oil brands. The first is taste. High-quality, pure oils do not taste fishy. Fresh oils are mild and sweet-tasting; rancid oils are strongly acrid and bitter. At home you can periodically puncture a capsule and squeeze a drop of oil onto your tongue to check out the taste. The color and clarity are also indications of freshness. As the oils age, they darken and become cloudy. A light color to the oil also assures the removal of the PCBs and heavy metals.

The "freezer test" is a good way to assess the EPA content of fish oils. Put a capsule in the freezer; if it congeals within a few hours, there is a high saturated fat content. The higher the saturated-fat content, the lower the EPA. Since most Americans are more deficient in the Omega-3s than the Omega-6s, it may be a good idea to replenish the Omega-3 reserves by consuming twice as much Omega-3 sources as Omega-6 for at least three to nine months. Afterward, the ratio can be balanced with equal amounts of Omega-6 as Omega-3. Here are some product supplements I routinely recommend to my clients that are balanced with the basic 1:1 ratio.

Product Name	Recommended Dosage
Super MAXEPA	1,000 mg
	1 twice daily with meals
Super-G 90	90 mg
	2 twice daily with meals
Female Formula	2 in morning with breakfast
or	
Male Formula	2 in morning with breakfast

Call Uni Key at 1-800-888-4353 to order.

Additional Fat Fighters

There are other vitamins that lower abnormally high fat levels, while others protect the essential fats from oxidation. Both niacin and vitamin C have been found to lower cholesterol levels in several clinical studies. Niacin is good for circulation and is a well-known blood vessel dilator. Vitamin C is a general overall blood vessel protector, which also supports the conversion of essential fatty acids into helpful prostaglandins. The English physician Constance Spittle has suggested that atherosclerosis results from long-term vitamin C deficiency, which allows cholesterol to accumulate in the artery walls. Of course, vitamin C, one of the body's best antioxidants, is also important in helping us deal with stress, increasing resistance, preventing collagen breakdown, and minimizing damage from environmental pollutants such as carbon monoxide, lead, cadmium, and mercury.

Cell Defense

The trace minerals selenium and zinc, as well as beta carotene and vitamins C and E, act as antioxidants to help protect vital tissues from the ravages of free radicals. Free radicals, you will remember, are produced by normal metabolic processes, as well as from exposure to radiation and to chemical carcinogens. Free radicals will attack sensitive cell membranes in DNA, causing a host of degenerative diseases. Antioxidants protect against these diseases by scavenging free radicals before they have a chance to do damage. These protective nutrients are found in whole grains, citrus fruits, and green leafy and deep yellow vegetables. The cruciferous family of cabbage, turnips, cauliflower, broccoli, and brussels sprouts are high in another cancer-combating family of substances called indoles.

Vitamin B-6 has supernutrient status as a fat metabolizer and heart disease preventive. Dr. Kilmer McCully,

formerly of the Harvard Medical School, believes that
B-6 can block the original injury to the arterial lining
caused by the toxic amino acid homocysteine. Vitamin
B-6 neutralizes the damaging homocysteine into a non-
toxic substance that the body can safely utilize. Foods
that are recommended vitamin B-6 sources include bananas, carrots, onion, kale, sweet potatoes, asparagus,
cauliflower, turnip greens, lentils, peas, and brewer's
yeast.

Garlic and Onions

Here are two popular vegetables that benefit lipid metabolism and are versatile favorites in the kitchen.
Practically every cuisine in the world makes use of the
food-enhancing and medicinal qualities of garlic and onions.

Garlic has been used since antiquity for its healing
benefits. During the Middle Ages its medicinal value was
prized against killer plagues. As recently as World War II,
it was used against typhus and dysentery. Garlic's strong
germicidal and strengthening actions have been recognized far into the twentieth century. It is very helpful
against yeast-fungus-related disorders. Dr. Michael J.
Wargovich of the Anderson Hospital and Tumor Institute
in Houston, Texas, reports that garlic oil may inhibit cancer growth in test animals.

The active substance in garlic is a volatile oil called
allicin, which has antibacterial and antifungal properties. Allicin is what gives garlic its unmistakable smell.
Allicin has been shown to be active against harmful bacteria without affecting friendly bacteria. In laboratory
culture studies, garlic has inhibited the growth of the
fungi *Candida albicans* and *Aspergillus niger*, two yeasts
that affect many allergic individuals.

Besides allicin, garlic also contains vitamins, and the
trace minerals vanadium and selenium (a potent antioxidant). Garlic's benefits have been known to help a wide

range of human maladies. High blood pressure, cardio-vascular disease, intestinal problems, liver trouble, and sinus conditions have all benefited from its use.

In the late 1960s, doctors began studying the fat-cutting properties of garlic. It proved to be a good food in combating high cholesterol and triglyceride levels. Clinical studies demonstrated its effectiveness in reducing platelet aggregation by cutting the stickiness of platelets, thereby reducing the tendency of blood to clot and preventing loss of blood flow through the arterial system. Garlic's numerous benefits in coronary artery disease are becoming well known.

In the '90s there is a lot of attention on garlic's ability to boost the immune system due to its rich sulfur content. In fact, according to Herbert F. Pierson, Ph.D., who is a research and development vice president for Preventive Nutrition Consultants, Inc., the real star ingredient in garlic may not be allicin at all but a chemical called S-allylcysteine. Animal studies have shown this substance to be effective in stopping the growth of breast tumors. Whether these effects are the same for humans is yet unknown, but S-allylcysteine looks promising.

In *Robert Crayhon's Nutrition Made Simple* (Evans, 1995), nutritionist Robert Crayhon provides a summary of garlic's many benefits:

- Garlic works as a natural antibiotic and reduces the number of harmful bacteria in the body.
- Garlic reduces blood cholesterol and triglyceride levels, and has been shown to limit the deposition of plaque on artery walls.
- Garlic has been shown to help the body eliminate parasites.
- Garlic reduces the amount of the yeast *Candida albicans* in the human GI tract and has been shown to be beneficial in fighting systemic yeast infections.
- Aged garlic extract has been shown to promote the growth of beneficial bacteria.
- Garlic has been shown to effectively lower blood sugar and be of significant benefit to diabetics.

- Garlic has been shown in population and laboratory studies to help prevent a wide variety of cancers.
- Garlic contains selenium, a cancer-preventing, immune-boosting, and anti-inflammatory nutrient.

Not to be overlooked, the lowly onion has also proved its worth in protecting the artery walls from blood clots and plaque buildup. The work of Dr. Victor Gurewich, professor of medicine at Tufts University and director of the vascular laboratory at St. Elizabeth's Hospital in Boston, has demonstrated that the juice of one yellow or white onion per day can dramatically raise the beneficial HDL cholesterol levels in the blood. The milder red onions seem not to have the same effect as the more pungent yellow or white varieties. Another prominent researcher, Dr. Arun Bordia, has lowered blood fats in coronary heart disease patients with both onions and garlic.

In cooking, garlic enjoys the distinction of being the second most used condiment in America (black pepper is the first). We love its flavoring in a wide variety of dishes from soups to salads to main courses. There are entire cookbooks devoted to garlic alone, and every year in Gilroy, California, there is a world-renowned garlic festival in which new and more innovative ways of eating the venerable "stinking rose" are created.

Studies of the onion show that cooking reduces its cholesterol-controlling ability. The same may apply to garlic, although aged garlic extract retains and even improves garlic's valuable properties. For everyday use, aged garlic extract may be the most beneficial.

11

FAT-BURNING NUTRIENTS

*Although overeating may be the cause of weight gain
in some individuals, many overweight people do not overeat.
These people are more likely the victims of
inefficient fat metabolism.*
—DALLAS CLOUATRE, PH.D.

I wish, like so many of you, that there really was one magic formula for weight loss that worked for everybody. The reality is that regular aerobic exercise plus a low-glycemic eating plan that includes the right fats and lean proteins provides the strongest foundation for fat burning and lasting weight loss. As you may remember from the chapter "Curbing Those Crazy Carbohydrates," it is wisest to choose basically carbohydrates that are lower on the Glycemic Index so that you will have sustained energy without a quick rise and fall of your blood sugar. When blood sugar is elevated too quickly, the hormone insulin is produced in abundance, and this process encourages both fat production and fat storage. High insulin levels in some individuals can also create a low blood sugar situation, or hypoglycemia, with symptoms such as irritability, weakness, and even dizziness and palpitations. The resulting low blood sugar creates more hunger and cravings for a quick fix, usually more sugar in the form of cookies, candy, and soda pop.

Yet there is some promising research that suggests

that certain nutrients boost the body's ability to burn fat. These nutrients include the mineral chromium, the amino acid L-Carnitine, the vitamins inositol and choline, and the enzyme lipase. While research about these supplements may not be totally conclusive, I believe that you can benefit from their use in conjunction with the right exercise and eating regimen.

The Chromium Connection

Chromium is probably the most highly publicized nutrient for its ability to increase body fat metabolism. Many of my clients report that although they have not lost much weight according to the bathroom scale, they have lost inches and have gone down several clothing sizes. Chromium is an essential trace mineral that is in very short supply in most diets. The primary reason may be that most of the soil in America today is lacking in chromium. The process of refining flour also depletes this mineral. It is found in the highest amounts in brewer's yeast, a supplemental food that is not in vogue because of its yeast-promoting potential. Other sources that contain lesser amounts include unprocessed whole grains, prunes, nuts, and black pepper. It is generally estimated that 9 out of 10 Americans are deficient in this most essential trace mineral.

Moreover, there is some indication that the high amounts of sugar eaten by most Americans can deplete the chromium supply in the body. Preliminary research suggests that the artificial sweetener aspartame may also be a chromium robber. Since aspartame is found in more than 3,000 foods, you never know how much you are actually ingesting. Diet sodas, the drink of choice these days in America, are usually sweetened with aspartame.

Chromium can also make insulin more effective in regulating blood sugar to the cell. In fact, the lack of chromium has been connected with a low sugar tolerance and even diabetes. Studies have shown that chromium supplementation results in lowered body fat, balanced blood sugar levels, increased muscle development, and the lessening of sugar cravings. It also has been shown to be helpful in lowering the bad LDL cholesterol and triglycerides while raising the good HDL cholesterol. Some indications have even pointed to chromium improving circulation by keeping the arteries clear. This has the added benefit of slowing down the aging process since the blood transports oxygen and nutrients to every part of the body. When the body is deprived of necessary oxygen and nutrients through blocked arteries, cell damage can occur.

How much chromium should you take? The National Academy of Sciences has suggested from 50 to 200 mcg. daily. Studies utilizing chromium for weight-loss purposes have used 200 or 400 mcg. daily. I believe that up to 400 mcg. daily can be helpful to some individuals.

L-Carnitine

Another nutritional strategy for combating abnormally high fat in the blood is the amino acid L-Carnitine. It is considered an effective fat burner because it transfers fatty acids into the mitochondria (the cells' fat-burning furnaces) and can lower cholesterol levels while elevating the good HDLs. L-Carnitine is also known to clean mitochondria of waste products as it enters these fat-burning furnaces to assist in the prevention of the production of free radicals, which are formed as a natural by-product when the mitochondria oxidize food for energy.

An L-Carnitine deficient body reveals itself through obesity, fatigue, muscle weakness, and elevated lipid levels. Some research suggests that certain types of obesity are caused by a genetic predisposition that causes the body to generate lower amounts of L-Carnitine than normal. Since the highest amounts of L-Carnitine are pro-

duced in the kidneys and liver, some problems with
those organs can also be hidden causes of lowered
L-Carnitine production. It is also directly related to the
function of the heart muscle and is deficient in damaged
heart tissues.

L-Carnitine is promoted as a product that enhances
"fat loss, weight loss, and muscle toning." It can be
found mainly in animal protein, especially lamb. This
amino acid can also be manufactured by the body from
proper amounts of iron, vitamins C and B-6, niacin, and
the amino acids methionine and lysine. Vegetarians, who
may not be getting enough methionine and lysine in
their diets, usually benefit from L-Carnitine supplementation.

I would suggest L-Carnitine in amounts of 50 mg. up
to 1,000 mg. daily, which most researchers recommend
for fat metabolism and fat burning. In my own experience, generally 250 mg. to 500 mg. a day produces
weight-loss results.

Choline and Inositol

Another popular fat-emulsifying substance is lecithin.
Lecithin is found in soy products and unprocessed vegetable oils and is very rich in the B-complex vitamins choline and inositol. These two B-vitamin members, in their
isolated forms, can help make lecithin in the liver. Both
choline and inositol can normalize total cholesterol, the
bad LDL cholesterol, and triglycerides. They are useful
in the treatment of high blood pressure too.

Inositol and choline are known as lipotropic factors. A
lipotropic factor aids the prevention of excess fat buildup
and assists in thinning or emulsifying fat so that it can be
easily moved through the bloodstream. This is especially
comforting when we are talking about the reduction of
that notorious fatty, orange peel–like substance called
cellulite because both choline and inositol are so efficient at fat management.

Lipotropics stimulate the thymus gland and can be helpful in preventing the formation of gallstones. Inositol, specifically, may help prevent nerve damage in diabetic neuropathy. It also aids in the transmission of nerve impulses and is considered a good memory stimulant. In addition, there are many herbal lipotropics that may be useful. These include turmeric, milk thistle, dandelion root, and Oregon grape root.

Lipase to the Rescue

The digestive enzyme lipase is also helpful in fat burning because it digests fat. Lipase is naturally produced by the pancreas, and it is also available in a plant enzyme form derived from fungi such as aspergillus, oryzae, and other similar species. This enzyme is naturally present in raw fats such as raw butter (unpasteurized butter), which may account for why the use of raw butter years ago in America did not make people gain weight. Lipase is absent in most of the fats that are currently used today because of cooking and pasteurization.

Primitive, isolated Eskimos were also great raw food eaters. They enjoyed raw meat as a central part of their diet and were not overweight. This may be because of the natural amounts of lipase in these foods. In *Enzyme Nutrition* (Avery, 1985), Dr. Edward Howell states that "there are dozens of reports in the periodic scientific literature during the last 50 years proclaiming that wherever the chemist finds fat in nature, he also finds the enzyme lipase."

Lipase can be taken as a supplemental fat-burning enzyme in amounts from 25 mg. to more than 200 mg. per capsule. Some individuals have reported good fat-burning results when taking from 3 to 5 capsules of lipase between meals. For fat reduction, lipase should be taken between meals because it can better attack fatty deposits in the body rather than digesting fats in the foods just eaten.

Herbal Magic

A word of caution is in order. There are certain herbs on the market that are being touted as the next generation of fat burners. Their claim to fat-burning fame is that they work by increasing thermogenesis in the body. Thermogenesis is the process of stoking the metabolic fire after eating or exercising. One of the main thermogenic herbs is Ephedra, or Ma huang (its Chinese name). Ephedra is one of the most controversial herbs today for good reason. While it can indeed jumpstart the metabolism, it has some rather serious side effects. Ephedra constricts blood vessels, elevates blood pressure, and raises the heart rate, all of which are decidedly contraindicated for individuals with diabetes, heart disease, hypertension, and kidney disease. While it does have benefit as a bronchodilator and decongestant, it is effective because it acts as a stimulant to the adrenal glands. The adrenals are responsible for the body's stress response and maintaining smooth blood sugar levels. Prolonged overuse of Ephedra can create adrenal exhaustion. Because of these factors, Ephedra cannot be recommended.

There are four additional herbs that are considered potent thermogenic agents: mate, guarana, kola nut, and white willow bark. The first three contain caffeine, which may initially give some people an energy boost but leave them exhausted and depleted in the long run. White willow bark, from which aspirin is derived, is high in salicylate. Its blood-thinning effect is therefore similar to that of aspirin. It is best in any case to check with your physician to make sure there are no secondary conditions that may be aggravated before taking any of these particular fat burners.

12

THE LOWDOWN ON FIBER

Fiber can make you free.
—JERRY VAN AMERONGEN
cartoonist

Fiber is the indigestible part of plant foods that we used to call "bulk" or "roughage." Because fiber is indigestible, it has no direct nutritional value, but it does have nutritional effects. Like essential fat, fiber gives the dieter a full feeling and many attendant health benefits. When fiber absorbs water and wells up in the intestines, you feel full and therefore satisfied with fewer calories. Other health bonuses from dietary fiber are a steady blood sugar level, cholesterol regulation, and better bowel elimination. These effects depend on the type of fiber eaten.

Dietary fiber can be divided into two types, soluble and insoluble. The water-soluble fibers from fruits, vegetables, peas, beans, and oats are rich in pectins and gums that slow down carbohydrate absorption, which stabilizes blood sugar levels. They are also believed to surround cholesterol molecules with a gellike coating that inhibits cholesterol absorption into the bloodstream. Water-soluble fibers may help to slow down digestion enough to enable the fat-digesting enzyme lipase to further break down fats before they are absorbed.

Insoluble fibers, from wheat bran, whole grains, and beans, assist in elimination. While they don't break down in water, they absorb water in the digestive tract, allowing waste materials to move out (transit) at a faster pace. Insoluble fiber is helpful in bowel disorders such as constipation and diverticular disease, in which weakened areas of the intestinal wall become inflamed. It may also protect against colon cancer by removing fat-soluble carcinogens. When fats and oils are eaten, the liver produces bile acids to break them down for further digestion in the intestines. Bile acids can become cancer causing if they remain in contact with the intestinal walls for too long. Fiber speeds up transit time so that noxious wastes are removed from the system quickly. This is why it is so important to have a good bowel movement at least once a day. Some authorities suggest two or three times a day. The point is that bowel wastes can decay and ferment and be reabsorbed into the bloodstream, thereby polluting cells, tissues, and organs.

Due to its coarseness, too much insoluble fiber may irritate the bowel—a problem not seen with the softer water-soluble fiber. Another problem with grain fiber, especially wheat bran, is that it can interfere with the absorption of minerals such as calcium, magnesium, iron, and zinc.

Here is a handy guide to finding the soluble fiber that works for you:

Where to Find Soluble Fiber

Food	Serving	Soluble Fiber (g)
GRAINS		
Oat bran	⅓ cup dry	2.0
All-Bran	⅓ cup	1.7
Oat bran muffin	1	1.6
Oatmeal	¾ cup, cooked	1.4
Rye bread	2 slices	0.6
Whole wheat bread	2 slices	0.5

Food	Serving	Soluble Fiber (g)
DRIED BEANS & PEAS		
Black-eyed peas	½ cup, cooked	3.7
Kidney beans	½ cup, cooked	2.5
Pinto beans	½ cup, cooked	2.3
Navy beans	½ cup, cooked	2.3
Lentils	½ cup, cooked	1.7
Split peas	½ cup, cooked	1.7
VEGETABLES		
Peas	½ cup, canned	2.7
Corn	½ cup, cooked	1.7
Sweet potato	1 baked	1.3
Zucchini	½ cup, cooked	1.3
Cauliflower	½ cup, cooked	1.3
Broccoli	½ cup, cooked	0.9
FRUIT		
Prunes	4	1.9
Pear	1	1.1
Apple	1	0.9
Banana	1	0.8
Orange	1	0.7

Source: Personal communication, Janet Tietyen, Research Dietician with Dr. James Anderson, University of Kentucky Medical Center.

Note: Researchers are still perfecting methods of analyzing the total and soluble fiber content of foods. These values may differ from Anderson's earlier values and those of other researchers.

Source: *Nutrition Action Health Letter*, December 1985.

Oat bran, which also contains very small amounts of GLA, is the hottest new water-soluble fiber these days. Studies conducted by Dr. James Anderson, chief of endocrinology at the University of Kentucky Medical Center, show that a regimen of oat bran reduced cholesterol levels by an average of 19 percent in a three-week period. The addition of oat bran, pectin, psyllium seed husks, and guar gum (a fiber from beans) have all proved helpful in lowering blood cholesterol levels in other clinical studies. Oat bran, however, is one of the easiest fiber sources to add to the diet. Because of its cholesterol-fighting ability, oat bran is a welcome addition to the diet of those with high serum cholesterol levels. It can be used as a breakfast cereal, a food thickener, or sprinkled over foods at any time of the day.

Dr. Denis Burkitt, a British surgeon who spent twenty years in Africa, is the pioneer of fiber research. While in Uganda, he observed that heart disease and cancer are virtually nonexistent among the rural Africans. Those who ate a coarse and fiber-full diet did not suffer, as do Americans, the diseases of constipation, hiatal hernia, and varicose veins. The Africans average a total of 25 grams of fiber per day, and with this increased bulk their stools have a shorter bowel transit time—approximately thirty hours instead of the seventy hours or more for the average American. A shorter transit time, as previously explained, means less time for bile wastes to decompose into toxic substances. Bacterial putrefaction is also minimized.

The average American diet contains about 10 grams of fiber. Levels of 25 to 40 grams would be more advisable for cleaner intestines, reduced hunger, and colon cancer prevention. High blood fats, as well as adult-onset diabetes, can also be managed by a high-fiber diet. Fiber slows down absorption of nutrients from the intestinal tract, resulting in more stable levels of blood sugar.

It is not necessary to count fiber grams as long as you are eating unrefined, unprocessed foods. Brown rice, for example, contains three times as much fiber as white rice; and a raw apple has twice as much fiber as an equivalent amount of applesauce. High-fiber foods such as beans, grains, and vegetables are rich in complex carbohydrates and are part of the *Beyond Pritikin* Diet.

Recognizing the fiber dilemma of modern day America, international food scientist Dr. Arnold Spicer, a contemporary of Dr. Denis Burkitt, has created a fiber-rich diet food. This food, called Spicer's Hunger Crunchers, contains 6 grams of fiber and is made with a special patented formula that enables the fiber to expand to a volume five times greater than the natural volume of wheat. The expansion technique breaks down the gluten component of the wheat, which allows those individuals with gluten sensitivities to enjoy Hunger Crunchers without the digestive difficulty that often accompanies other wheat-based foods.

The expanded Hunger Crunchers, enjoyed as a complete food in itself, absorbs liquids and expands the muscle lining of the stomach so that hunger is delayed. Satiety is reached with as little as 100 calories per bag because of this process. Although Hunger Crunchers contain corn oil, the corn oil is not heated during the processing of the food. The oil is also protected from oxidation by a special packaging material. Considering these factors, the production is more nutritionally sound than most other snack foods on the market.

The technology to create high-fiber snack foods has already been developed. Like Walnut Acres in total food processing, Spicer's International is a forerunner in nutritious convenience foods. Hunger Crunchers are available in eight flavors and can be found in General Nutrition stores, drugstores, and convenience stores all over the United States.

13

NEW LIGHT ON FITNESS

*Few seem conscious that there is such
a thing as physical morality.*
—HIPPOCRATES

Any diet book worth its weight (loss) has to consider exercise as a way to burn additional calories. This part of the *Beyond Pritikin* Diet plan may well be the easiest part to follow. There are really no excuses in this area because the exercise prescription stays away from taxing anatomical activity such as jogging or heavy workouts. Instead, the preferred exercises are dancing, swimming, cycling, and walking with walking the Number One choice. Remember, though, to consult with your physician before beginning any exercise program.

The important aspect these three forms of exercise have in common is that they are all aerobic. Exercise that increases the body's use of oxygen is considered aerobic. The benefits from aerobic exercise include:

- Conditioning of heart, lungs, and blood vessels
- Firming and toning of muscles
- Increased coordination and flexibility of joints
- Improvements in circulation and general endurance

Medical research has shown that individuals who are more active suffer fewer heart attacks. They are also more likely to survive a heart attack. The *Journal of the American Medical Association* has reported that with regular aerobic exercise, high blood pressure can be reduced in mildly hypertensive people. Because modern lifestyles have made us increasingly sedentary, we need to schedule our exercise on a regular basis.

It is important to include some form of aerobic activity at least three to five times a week for a period of 20 to 30 minutes. To make sure your exercise is effective, it is wise to check your target heart rate (THR). Reaching your THR for at least 20 minutes is a goal of aerobic exercise.

To calculate your maximum heart rate, subtract your age from 220. Your target heart rate is 65 percent to 85 percent of your maximum heart rate. For example, if you are 40 years old, your maximum heart rate would be 180 (220 − 40 = 180). Your low-end THR is 127 (65 percent of 180) and your high-end THR is 153 (85 percent of 180). When beginning an exercise program, start at the lower value and work up slowly. It is important to allow the heart muscle time to strengthen and adjust to each increase in heart rate. In overweight and unconditioned individuals, this may take as long as two years.

To measure your heart rate, take your pulse on your wrist or neck immediately after at least 20 minutes of exercise. Count for 15 seconds and multiply by 4. For example, if you count 32 heartbeats in 15 seconds, your heart rate is 128 beats per minute. This is well within the boundaries of your target heart rate.

It is important to remember that muscle tissue burns more energy than fat tissue. Pound for pound, muscle burns five times as many calories as other tissue. The most effective exercise is weight lifting or resistance training because of muscle buildup that burns excess calories. The greater the amount of muscle tissue, the higher the metabolic rate. A further bonus of exercise is that it affects body metabolism for up to fifteen hours after you stop doing the exercise itself. Exercise can also suppress appetite for several hours. If you exercise before dinner you will eat less and relieve the tension that builds up during the day. And if you exercise after dinner, you burn up to 15 percent more calories than you do when exercising on an empty stomach.

Walking is your best bet because, of all the sports, it is most easily accessible to most people at most times of the year. Walking is preferred over running because running imposes a great deal of stress on the knees and skeletal system. Injuries to joints and tendons are common because with each stride while running, the impact is increased to four times the body's weight. In women, this impact can have devastating effects on the fragile pelvic bones, especially in postmenopausal women (with tendencies toward osteoporosis).

Brisk, vigorous walking burns just as many calories per mile as does running. It may even provide better muscle toning than running because, when walking a mile, more steps are taken than when running a mile. When you walk, try to move your whole body vigorously. New research reports that exercise in which both the arms and the legs are actively moving is a better fat burner than exercise in which only the legs are involved. This is why cross-country skiing is so highly rated for its calorie-burning benefits, as well as the NordicTrack and stationary rowing machines. So get into it and move all of your body.

Walk wherever and whenever you can. The only other requirement is that walking be done outside during the daytime. Natural light, like essential fat, is an endangered nutrient in which many of us are deficient. We spend too much time indoors under incandescent and fluorescent lights that prevent natural full-spectrum light from entering our eyes. Even the glass in our office windows, automobiles, eyeglasses, and contact lenses blocks the beneficial ultraviolet rays from natural daylight. Light entering the eyes influences the master glands such as the pineal, which influences mood and behavior, and the pituitary, which controls all the other glands of the endocrine system. We need the entire full spectrum of natural sunlight for complete health. Inadequate exposure to natural illumination can induce a form of depression known as "seasonal affective disorder" (SAD). SAD has been shown to result from diminished exposure to natural light as the days grow shorter.

You should walk briskly for at least 30 minutes outside, without sunglasses, regular glasses, or contact lenses if possible to allow the sunlight to reach the retina of the eye. When walking, get your heart pumping at your target heart rate and try to maintain that pace for 20 minutes. If you are in an office and can't exercise during working hours, try to take some of your lunch or coffee breaks outside in the sun, and take off your glasses!

Dancing is another good exercise. The low-impact aerobic dancing, square dancing, and fast-moving ballroom dancing are all enjoyable and fun. Home exercise videotapes now feature low-intensity workouts that are also good movers. More important, they are safer for people who are out of shape or overweight than the earlier high-intensity type because they are paced and build endurance slowly but surely.

Swimming is a very popular and recommended exercise. Because the body weight is suspended in water, every muscle in the body can be exercised without strain. To really condition the muscles, you might try poolwalking. At the shallow end of the pool, walk from one side to the other, which has the effect of dragging the legs through the water. This provides a beneficial workout for all the leg muscles.

Bicycling is also a beneficial body conditioner. Outside, for full-spectrum light, and out of traffic, for full-spectrum safety, bicycling provides good cardiovascular exercise. The bicycle seat should be as high as possible while still keeping your knees slightly bent at full extension. The gears should be as low as possible to enable easy, rapid pedaling. If you climb a lot of hills, use the low gears on a ten-speed bike. If you use a stationary bike, take it outdoors or put it in front of an open window where sunlight can reach your eyes.

Of course, there are many other suitable aerobic exercises that stimulate the heart and burn calories. By all means, if your favorite activity is tennis, racquetball, skipping rope, rowing, cross-country skiing, roller skating, or even stair climbing, then continue it on a regular basis. Whenever you enjoy what you do, you are more likely to continue to do it.

14

CHEMISTRY IN THE KITCHEN

Most health problems begin in the kitchen.
—PAUL DUDLEY WHITE, M.D.

Now it's time to turn to the practical issues. That is, what you should eat and how the food should be prepared for optimum health. Let's review and summarize some basic tenets of the *Beyond Pritikin* Diet. Here are the Prime Contenders:

Prime Contenders

- Expeller-pressed crude or unrefined oils

  For salad: Safflower, flaxseed, sunflower, sesame, corn, walnut, almond, hazelnut, peanut, canola oil, extra virgin olive, and virgin olive.

  For cooking: Peanut, canola oil, coconut oil, extra virgin and virgin olive, high oleic safflower and sunflower oil.

Note: Shelled raw nuts and seeds from which the above are derived are not a reliable good-fat source because they are generally rancid from exposure to heat, air, and light. They are best bought unshelled in the raw state and then "home toasted" before eating. Commercially roasted nuts have been heated at excessively high temperatures, which hastens rancidity. More information about how to purchase, store, and prepare these foods is included under "Desirable Cooking Methods," p. 127, and "Stocking and Storing the Staples," p. 141. I suggest that nuts and seeds be used primarily as condiments.

Sesame seed butter is an unusually stable nut butter that resists rancidity. It is particularly high in calcium and the two amino acids methionine and tryptophan, which are usually deficient in most vegetable proteins.

- **Cold-water fish**   Salmon, mackerel, tuna, sablefish, herring, anchovies, sardines, rainbow trout, Alaska king and blue crab, oysters, bass, catfish, halibut, cod, shrimp, pilchard, flounder, haddock, and bluefish.

- **Fresh-water fish**   Trout and crappie.

- **Fiber**   Oats, apples, peas, prunes, and legumes such as black-eyed peas, all beans such as kidney, pinto, and navy, and agar-agar seaweed gelatin.

- **Vegetables, fruits, and whole grains**   All varieties, especially antioxidant-rich leafy greens, deep yellow vegetables; cruciferous family of broccoli, cabbage, brussels sprouts, cauliflower, and turnips rich in indoles or cancer inhibitors.

- **Water**   Eight glasses a day keeps the system washing away.

- **Supplements**   GLA, EPA; the support vitamins niacin (B-3), B-6, C, and E; antioxidant beta carotene; the minerals zinc, magnesium, and selenium.

- **Aerobic exercise**   30-minute walk at vigorous pace outside in sunlight or equivalent aerobic activity like dancing, swimming, bicycling, Nordic-Track, or stair climbing.

Prime Offenders

These foods are most affected by heat, oxidation, hydrogenation, or homogenization and should be avoided.

- **Trans or damaged fats**   Margarine, shortening, and baked goods containing hydrogenated oils such as breads, cookies, cakes, and taco shells; commercial vegetable oils; commercial peanut butter; all fried foods, primarily french fries.

- **Homogenized fats**   Full-fat and low-fat (2 percent) homogenized cow's milk and dairy product derivatives such as cheese and yogurt.

- **Oxidized cholesterol**   Dried milk, dried eggs, dried custard mixes, smoked fish, aged cheese.

These foods biochemically sabotage the metabolism.

- **White refined sugar**   Cakes, cookies, candies, pies, and soft drinks. Eliminate and eat only natural sources from fresh fruit.

- **Alcohol**   Use only in cooking (the alcohol burns off and the flavor remains).

These foods can be harmful only *without* the balancing EFAs.

• Saturated fats	All animal fats, particularly beef tallow, and palm oil (used in some fast food preparation); coconut oil (used in nondairy creamers) and palm oil both found in shortening, some soups, whipped topping, some frostings, frozen entrees, cookies, and snack foods. Palm kernel oil is an ingredient in carob candies.

Nutritional Bombshells

As you now know from the preceding chapters, it isn't the fat itself that is a problem, but what we do *to* the fat. When I first discovered this, I began to explore every facet of food, from selection to handling to storage to cooking methods, and food combinations and cooking utensils. I uncovered some surprising nutritional insights that discredit many accepted nutritional truths. Now we know:

- A high-carbohydrate diet or a high grain intake may be weight promoting and energy draining.
- Cooking with polyunsaturated oils is more dangerous than using small amounts of saturated fat, such as butter.
- Homogenized milk may be an underlying cause of heart disease and needs more investigation.
- Cholesterol-free margarines can be devastating to health.
- Exercising in daylight is distinctly more beneficial than exercising indoors.

But there is more surprising information that is covered in chapter 15, "The *Beyond Pritikin* Diet Master Strategy." There you will discover:

- If you cook with aluminum, what you're cooking in may have as much influence over your health as what you are cooking.
- Frozen fruits and vegetables can be more nutritious than their fresh counterparts.
- Rare is rarely the most healthy way to cook fish or meat.
- Red meats have a very important place in a well-balanced diet.

The Life in Your Food

Cooking is actually a form of chemistry. It can either protect or destroy food value and nutrients. Canning, freezing, storage, and cooking all create vitamin and mineral loss that can affect good health.

In canning, for example, there can be a 40 to 60 percent loss of vitamins. While freezing retains more vitamins, there still may be up to a 45 percent loss in the blanching process necessary to neutralize enzymes.

From the time of harvesting to shipping, warehouse storage of lettuce, spinach, and potatoes can result in a loss of up to 50 percent of their vitamin C. Because of the time elapsed from harvesting to the supermarket shelf, fresh produce can be less nutritious in certain cases than even the frozen variety. Furthermore, if the fresh produce is stored at too high a temperature in shipping or storage, additional loss of thiamin (vitamin B-1), riboflavin (vitamin B-2), niacin (vitamin B-3), and vitamin C can result. Fresh produce always should be stored on ice or in an area cooler than room temperature.

Cooking with too much water depletes vitamins B and C, while using baking soda to keep vegetables green is another potent destroyer of vitamin C.

Food Follies

The way in which food is cooked and handled can mean the difference between health and disease. Frying and prolonged broiling of meat and fish produce genetic changes in bacteria known to cause cancer in test animals. Food-poisoning bacteria like salmonella are found in raw meats, eggs, poultry, fish, shellfish, and milk. These foods may taste just fine but still be infected. All cutting boards, knives, and plates used in the preparation of raw meat and poultry must be thoroughly washed before reusing them for cooked food. Pathogenic organisms can be transferred from infected food to cooked foods to you. The result can be those flulike symptoms that last a few hours to a few days, now so common that people don't even consult a doctor when they occur. Even worse, food poisoning can cause chronic joint problems such as arthritis and other rheumatoid diseases, according to the FDA's Dr. Douglas Archer, director of the Microbiology division.

The FDA believes that in 1985 about 4 million Americans were infected with salmonella: 35,000 were hospitalized. But who knows how many people actually had salmonella in their dinner and never knew what hit them? The USDA estimates that 30 percent of all poultry in this country is salmonella-infected due to the processing of chicken. Some researchers suggest that the number is actually much closer to 60 percent.

I have designed the *Beyond Pritikin* Diet Master Menu Plan for good eating and healthful food preparation. All foods you will be eating are considered. You will learn the best ways to select, prepare, serve, and store them. Remember, your kitchen is your personal laboratory. Observing simple rules of chemistry in food preparation can mean a great health savings not only in terms of greater nutritional value, but in the avoidance of routine illnesses that start in the kitchen.

Nutritional Savvy

The first rule is that heat, light, soaking in water, and extended exposure to air can destroy valuable vitamins as well as the beneficial fats. High temperatures and oxidation can alter fatty acid bonds and create rancidity. Amino acids (the building blocks of protein) become unusable by the body when protein foods are overheated, as in frying. An innocent-looking piece of fried chicken, for example, has not only whopping numbers of extra calories, but its protein is less valuable.

Vegetables cut long before they're used, salad-bar style, have lost many nutrients.

The B vitamins are especially vulnerable to heat and light. Riboflavin (vitamin B-2) is the most sensitive to light, which is why many dairies now use cardboard cartons instead of glass bottles to contain milk, a good source of riboflavin. (Deficiency symptoms include cracks around the corners of the mouth and eyes, eye burning, pupil dilation, oily skin, and fatigue.)

Both vitamins B and C are water-soluble and easily lost from produce soaked longer than one hour. The lesson in all of this:

1. Low, slow cooking.
2. The less water touches the food, the better for vitamins.
3. Prepare food right before you cook it.

Temperature Control

Exposure to room-temperature air can oxidize the cholesterol in animal foods, causing altered blood chemistry. No animal food, such as meat, fish, cheese, milk, eggs, or butter, should be left standing outside the refrigerator for more than two hours.

A simple rule always to keep in mind is: Keep hot foods hot (140 degrees and above) and cold foods cold (40 degrees and lower). See the chart on temperature of food for control of bacteria.

Most of us take our refrigerators for granted. Under-

Temperature of Food For Control of Bacteria

°C	°F	
121	250	Canning temperatures for low-acid vegetables, meat, and poultry in pressure canner.
116	240	
		Canning temperatures for fruits, tomatoes, and pickles in water-bath canner.
100	212	
		Cooking temperatures destroy most bacteria. Time required to kill bacteria decreases as temperature is increased.
74	165	
		Warming temperatures prevent growth but allow survival of some bacteria.
60	140	
		Some bacterial growth may occur. Many bacteria survive.
52	120	
		DANGER ZONE. Temperatures in this zone allow rapid growth of bacteria and production of toxins by some bacteria. (Foods in this temperature zone should not be held for more than 2 or 3 hours.)
16	60	
		Some growth of food poisoning bacteria may occur.
4	40	
0	32	Cold temperatures permit slow growth of some bacteria that cause spoilage. (Raw meats should be used within 5 days, ground meat, poultry, and fish within 2 days.
		Freezing temperatures stop growth of bacteria, but may allow bacteria to survive.
−18	0	

Adapted from *Keeping Food Safe to Eat*, Home and Garden Bulletin No. 162, U.S. Department of Agriculture, 1970.

standing how this appliance can help you in properly caring for food is a cornerstone for good nutrition.

1. Adjust your refrigerator temperature to 40 degrees.
2. The freezer should be kept at zero degrees.
3. Get a thermometer if your freezer indicates only HIGH or LOW temperature levels.
4. Check frost levels. If more than one-quarter inch of frost builds up, the cooling process is slowed down. It is time to defrost.

Other Helpful Hints

• Do not stack foods on top of one another in the refrigerator. Circulation of cold air is important to prevent spoilage.

• Store perishables where you can see them. Fish gravies and meat broths should be used up in two days.

The following indicators on the oven or stove translate into temperatures:

- • Warm   = 125 to 200 degrees
- • Boiling = 212 to 300 degrees
- • Frying   = 350 degrees and above

When food is kept over a long period of time, it should be held in the oven at 140 degrees or higher to prevent bacteria from growing. Get a meat thermometer to accurately measure the temperature of food.

Selection of Vegetables and Fruits

Follow these guidelines to get the most nutritional mileage from your food:

Select fresh vegetables, preferably locally grown. This is a first step to ensure that nutrients have not been lost during shipping and storing. Frozen is the next-best choice. Many vegetables and fruits are frozen at the peak of ripeness in their growing season, so taste can be exceptionally flavorful in certain vegetables such as peas, corn, and lima beans. Just remember that if your vegetables are frozen (and this goes for frozen food in general, by the way), thaw them in the refrigerator and then cook them immediately to prevent bacteria from spreading.

Hydroponic (soilless) growing of fruits, vegetables, and herbs is a promising agricultural development. In a greenhouse environment plants are fed by a flow of water rich in essential nutrients. Growth is enhanced, and the food produced is often much higher in vitamins and minerals than that of soil-fed plants. Yet, the long-term effects of consumption by humans has not been assessed—there may be other essential factors from the soil that cannot be duplicated in a soilless environment. These effects are electromagnetic and cannot be measured by conventional science, so the verdict is not yet in.

Remember that moldy, soggy, or discolored patches on celery, broccoli, or cauliflower are a sign of deterioration. Root vegetables with wilted or watery leaves should be avoided. Do not buy potatoes that are green or sprouting. This indicates the presence of a toxin called solanine. Carrots with hairy roots are also nutrient-deprived.

Remember that fully matured vegetables have the most nutrition of all. Sweet red peppers, for example, have 7.5 times more vitamin A than immature green peppers. Ripe red tomatoes contain 3.5 times more vitamin A than green tomatoes.

Certain varieties of produce give you better nutrition for your money. Romaine lettuce, for example, has more than twice the iron, calcium, and vitamin C of iceberg.

Successful Vegetable Storage

• Do not store vegetables with fruits. The natural gas that fruits produce when ripening—ethylene—can make vegetables deteriorate.

• Store vegetables in lower bins away from the freezer section to prevent crystallization. Store dry and wash right before use, unless you are using a Clorox bath to cleanse all produce before storing (see p. 149). Excess moisture encourages mold growth.

• Store greens leafy side down in a twist-tied plastic bag. Before closing the bag, retain a little air inside to keep the greens from wilting.

• Store root vegetables such as potatoes, onions, hard-skinned squash, and yams in a cool, dry pantry (50–70 degrees) away from direct sunlight.

Like vegetables, certain fruits are better health buys. Pink grapefruit are 50 times higher in vitamin A than white grapefruit. Oranges from California are 34 percent higher in vitamin C than Florida oranges. Avocados grown in California are 15 percent higher in fat, which may account for their superior flavor, than those from Florida.

Many frozen fruits are actually a better buy than the fresh variety. Frozen berries—blueberries, raspberries, strawberries, blackberries, and boysenberries—are generally uniformly sweet and flavorful. Fresh berries, by the time they reach the market, are often overripe and spoiled from handling. Those at the bottom of the basket are sometimes crushed and inedible. Mold forms almost instantly on a crushed berry.

Successful Fruit Storage

Store fruits dry and wash right before eating. Unripened fruits such as melons, bananas, avocados, peaches, plums, pears, and tomatoes can be kept in a dry, cool pantry away from direct sunlight. Lemons, limes, grapefruit, and oranges can be kept in the pantry, too. Fully ripened fruit should be kept in the refrigerator bins. Berries should be stored covered.

Vegetable Preparation and Cooking

Limit cutting, peeling, and soaking of vegetables. Exposure to air, light, and water robs essential vitamins and minerals. Cook over low heat and keep the lid on during cooking.

Vegetables can be prepared by cooking in a covered pan, Crockpot, or stainless steel steamer. They also can be prepared by poaching or sautéing, in a very small amount of virgin olive oil, canola oil, peanut oil, or butter. Other vegetable oils produce dangerous free radicals when heated, so use the more stable olive or peanut oil or butter (one tablespoon) for cooking.

Never bake vegetables uncovered unless you are using a microwave oven. Dry heat evaporates natural juices, where most of the vitamins and minerals are contained. When baking vegetables (and this goes for baked potatoes, especially), bake in a covered container at 350 degrees or below. To obtain the crispy skin of baked potatoes, uncover for the last ten to fifteen minutes of cooking.

Fruit Preparation and Cooking

Ultimately, it is more important that fruit be fully ripened than whether it is fresh, frozen, or canned in its own juices. Frozen and canned fruit in its own juice are harvested at the peak of ripeness and so are good fruit choices. Unripened fruit creates gas, bloating, and much digestive discomfort.

Fruit fibers are more easily broken down in cooking than are vegetable fibers. Fruit sugar therefore becomes more concentrated in the bloodstream without the fiber to regulate its release. This is why raw, ripe fruit is more desirable than cooked fruit for those who want to control their blood sugar levels.

There are two fruits, however, in which the health value is actually enhanced by cooking. These are blueberries and blackberries. These fruits, in their raw state, contain a thiamine-destroying enzyme. Thiamine (vitamin B-1) is essential for the nervous system and is known as the "morale vitamin." When the berries are cooked (or frozen), the enzyme is deactivated.

"Baked" rather than "raw" apples are better tolerated by people who have digestive problems.

Fish, Fowl, and Meat

Whether purchased fresh (which is preferred) or frozen, all flesh foods must be cooked. If frozen, they should be thawed in the refrigerator and then cooked immediately after defrosting. Both fowl and meat thaw at the rate of one pound per hour. Again, all utensils as well as hands that come in contact with raw fish, fowl, and meat must be thoroughly washed to prevent bacterial infection.

Cooking temperatures must reach 160 to 180 degrees to kill disease-causing bacteria and other organisms. Most such organisms are destroyed at 140 degrees, but to ensure that all parts of the food are thoroughly heated, cooking at 160 to 180 degrees guarantees a safety margin against the heartier "bugs."

Undercooked, rare, or raw flesh foods can carry the eggs of such parasites as tapeworm (in fish and beef), liver flukes (beef), and the parasites that cause toxoplasmosis (beef and lamb). These organisms can seriously and chronically affect nutrient absorption and overall health. Parasitic disease is hard to trace, so symptoms such as cramps, diarrhea, constipation, and muscular aches and pains can go on for years.

Raw flesh foods such as sushi (raw fish), steak tartare, and carpaccio (raw beef) are definitely *not* recommended. Fish should be cooked so that all parts flake easily. Beef should be cooked to medium (160 degrees), and poultry should contain no pink areas and the joints should be easily movable.

Successful Meat Storage

• Refrigerate or freeze all raw meat, fish, and poultry immediately to prevent bacteria growth.

• When you refrigerate, choose the coldest section nearest the freezer, and cook as soon as possible.

• An uncooked chicken can remain only up to two days before spoilage sets in. Cooked chicken lasts up to five days.

• Cooked meats last longer when stored with sauces or gravies containing vegetables such as onions, peppers, potatoes, and tomatoes, which are high in the antioxidant vitamins A, E, and C. The fat in the meat can combine with oxygen in the refrigerator, allowing rancidity to set in. The vegetables protect the meat.

Help Line

The U.S. Department of Agriculture operates a Meat and Poultry Hotline at (800) 535-4555, Monday through Friday. Experts can answer everything you ever wanted to know about handling meat and fowl.

Shellfish

Like other fish, all shellfish should be cooked. Uncooked shellfish such as clams and oysters carry hepatitis A and Norwalk virus. These viruses can easily be mistaken for the flu because their symptoms are similar. Raw shellfish from contaminated waters offer more serious—and sometimes deadly—problems. Furthermore, there is an enzyme present in raw clams and oysters that destroys thiamine (vitamin B-1). Steam clams for an optimum of six minutes.

Seeds, Peanuts, Nuts, Beans, Egg Whites, and Potatoes

Although these seemingly random foods don't appear to have much in common, they do in one respect: they all should be cooked for maximum health benefits. This group contains enzyme inhibitors that interfere with proper digestion, creating gas, heartburn, and gastrointestinal problems. The enzyme inhibitors are destroyed by cooking. In the case of seeds, nuts, and beans, the enzyme inhibitors can also be deactivated by sprouting. First soak for six hours, then sprout. Toasting is another way to deactivate the inhibitors. All seeds and nuts, and peanuts (technically a legume) can be "home roasted" in the oven (see p. 128).

Always cook your eggs and potatoes. Raw egg whites contain avidin, a protein that inhibits biotin (a vitamin of the vitamin B complex family) absorption. When you cook eggs for thirty seconds or more, the avidin is destroyed, thus allowing full release of biotin for the body.

Many people soak grains before eating. Soaking increases digestibility of wheat, rye, oats, and barley (the higher-gluten grains) without digestive upsets. Simply soak in water overnight and cook the next morning.

Desirable Cooking Methods

Stir sautéing   Cooking in small amounts of liquid or oil (water, peanut oil, canola oil, virgin olive oil, vegetable broth, or defatted chicken broth) at medium heat. Do not use polyunsaturated vegetable oils such as safflower or corn, which are extremely heat sensitive.

Steaming
Cooking over boiling water in a large or small steamer pot, stainless steel folding basket, or Chinese-style tiered bamboo steamer. Steaming preserves nutrients, color, and texture, and accentuates flavor while keeping in moisture. The leftover liquid can be used for soups or stir sautéing.

When cooking highly concentrated carbohydrate foods such as sweet potatoes and yams, steam instead of baking. The baking temperatures precipitate the natural sugar into a caramelized substance, changing the complex carbohydrate into a simple sugar.

Broiling
Cooking in a broiler with overhead direct heat. Keep the oven door open. Nutrients are destroyed when the oven door is closed because the food dehydrates when surrounded by dry heat.

Toasting
Cooking in the oven at baking temperatures below 300 degrees. Seeds and nuts should be "home toasted." Low-level heating deactivates the enzyme inhibitors. Heating above 300 degrees, common in commercial roasting practices, changes the oil from the natural cis form to the damaged trans form.

Baking
Cooking in covered utensils with minimum liquid to retain moistness.

Microwave
Microwave cooking heats the food by friction of the food's molecules. This is

opposite to other cooking methods, in which the outside air surrounding the food must first be heated before the food begins to cook. Cooking in a microwave does not make the food radioactive despite the common misconception. Microwave cooking may even protect vitamins and minerals better than conventional methods but care must be taken with certain foods. Because microwaves do not cook uniformly, rotating meats such as chicken and pork is necessary to protect against salmonella in the chicken and trichina in the pork.

When cooking meat or fish in a microwave oven, be sure to check the internal temperature in many different places. Fish must be heated to an internal temperature of 140°F for at least five minutes. Beef, to at least 160°F, lamb, veal, and pork to 170°F.

Food prepared in a microwave may not be as visually appealing or appetizing because it does not brown after cooking. Convection microwave ovens or ovens with special browning features can achieve a more finished food look.

Undesirable Cooking Methods

Avoid frying

Frying is an all too common technique used in coffeeshops and restaurants, as well as in the preparation of popular snack foods such as doughnuts, potato chips, and many bakery products.

Tasty as these foods are, overheating of polyunsaturated oils produces more free radicals than overheating of saturated fats. These foods should carry the Surgeon General's warning. Frying meat, fish, or chicken also makes the protein bond indigestible.

When palm or coconut oil is used for frying, there are many less free radicals formed because these oils are saturated. Too much of the saturated oils present another problem, though, because their presence can block the natural cis linoleic from transforming to the vital GLA. Plus, harmful toxins that have been associated with cancer are produced no matter what source of fat is used when heated at high temperatures (350 degrees) or reheated with the same oil source. When you do fry, do not reheat the oil; throw it out.

Avoid browning or charring or charcoal grilling

The oxidative reaction of charcoal grilling (a combination of browning and charring) is toxic and can be carcinogenic. Further, food soaks up added chemicals from the charcoal briquettes. One piece of barbecued meat may be the carcinogenic equivalent of sixty cigarettes. It would be wise to cut off any burned, charred, or blackened portions of meat. Charcoal broiling should be avoided.

Gas grilling—with adequate ventilation—is acceptable if there is no sensitivity to hydrocarbons, the toxic byproducts of gas combustion.

Avoid
pressure
cooking

The temperatures are too high and destroy vitamins. This method is suitable, however, for canning foods at home.

More fuel for
thought

It is better to use electric rather than gas ranges and ovens for your cooking needs. The pilot lights and burners on gas ranges can release low levels of carbon monoxide and nitrous dioxide that often go undetected because they are invisible and odorless. Undiagnosable psychiatric conditions have even been traced to natural gas leakages. Symptoms such as dizziness, headache, confusion, chronic fatigue, insomnia, and respiratory problems can have their roots in unrecognized gas emissions. If you suspect that you may be suffering from "indoor pollution," have your local gas company come to your house and check for a gas leak.

Essential Utensils

- Stainless steel

Heavy stainless steel waterless cookware cooks food in a vacuum seal in its own juices. This is more expensive than the regular stainless, which is also desirable, but can protect mineral and vitamin content more thoroughly.

- Enamel
- Corning Ware
- Glass

Purists beware. Because glass and Pyrex do let in light, they may allow small amounts of light-sensitive riboflavin to become depleted.

- Pyrex
- Iron

The extra iron picked up from cooking is good for you. When spaghetti sauce, for example, is cooked in iron pots, it contains six times more iron than when made in ceramic cookware.

Baking equipment should be heavy-duty tin or black steel. Glass, stainless steel bowls, cling-free plastic wrap, or plastic bags (the kind used in the produce section of the supermarket) are best for food storage and freezing. There is also a hypoallergenic cellophane bag now available at health food stores for more sensitive individuals. The above mentioned materials do not dissolve into the food.

I personally use and recommend Royal Prestige Cookware. Food is cooked by the minimum moisture method at 180°F—the temperature that kills germs, bacteria (like E. coli), and parasites, not vitamins and minerals. Royal Prestige is available through Uni Key at 1-800-888-4353.

Essential Utensil Alert

It may seem as though we live in an ultracivilized, totally sanitary environment, but in fact there are some potentially dangerous situations common to almost every American kitchen. They're all easy to remedy, so give some thought to the following:

• *Throw out all cracked dishes.*
Bacteria can live in the cracks of cups and plates. These bacteria will mix with hot beverages or foods, creating digestive problems.

• *Replace or Clorox wooden cutting and chopping boards.*
Again, bacteria can live in the cracks of wooden blocks. Use a Lucite chopping board, or give your wooden board a Clorox rinse (use approximately ten drops of Clorox to a quart of water).

- *Avoid unlined copper pots and pans.*

Copper can contaminate acidic food and destroy vitamin C, and is antagonistic to zinc. Brass containers usually contain copper, so do not store food in them.

- *Eliminate aluminum and aluminum foil.*

No food or drink, especially acidic foods that are tomato based, should be cooked or covered in aluminum or aluminum foil.

Aluminum can affect digestion by destroying the protein-digestive enzyme pepsin in the stomach. It also hampers the body's utilization of calcium, magnesium, and phosphorous as well as vitamin A. Impaired memory and motor coordination as well as Alzheimer's disease and osteoporosis have been linked to systemic aluminum toxicity. The kidneys, brain, and gastrointestinal tract are the target areas where aluminum accumulates and can cause problems.

This metal is also found in antacids such as Maalox, Mylanta, Gelusil, Di-Gel, and Rolaids. Studies have shown that even small amounts of antacids can inhibit intestinal absorption of fluoride and phosphorus, causing increased elimination of calcium. Since calcium loss is a prime factor in osteoporosis—the bone-thinning disease—the answer is not more calcium but less aluminum.

Pain relievers such as Arthritis-Strength Bufferin, Ascriptin, Bufferin, Pabirin, and Vanquish contain aluminum.

- *Parchment paper: the foil to aluminum foil.*

Instead of aluminum foil for cooking and reheating, use parchment paper. It is available in most health food stores and is excellent for retaining flavor because the food cooks in its own juice. Made from wood pulp, it is a healthy alternative to metals and plastics. Ideal for vegetables and fish (as New Orleans cooks have known for years), parchment paper can be used for baking and poaching. The food is placed on top of a moistened parchment sheet, then the corners are gathered up and tied securely.

- *Aluminum-proof the kitchen.*

Check all steamers, measuring cups, spoons, bread pans, and cookie sheets. These items can all be safely replaced by Pyrex, stainless steel, or dairy tin (an old-fashioned baking material).

It may also be a good idea to replace aluminum-containing baking powders, as well as deodorants and antiperspirants, to generally reduce exposure to aluminum buildup, which accumulates in the body and can progressively deposit in the organs, muscles, and tissues. Aluminum, because of its astringent quality, irritates mucous membranes in the gastrointestinal tract.

- *The great outdoors.*

When camping out, remember to take extra care with certain foods. Ground meat is more subject to oxidation than whole meat. Cook it as soon as possible.

Do not drink water from streams and lakes because many have become contaminated with microorganisms such as *Giardia lamblia* and Cryptosporidium, which make their home in the gastrointestinal tract and the gallbladder. These amoebalike one-celled animals can cause chronic diarrhea and a whole host of health problems such as chronic fatigue, irritable bowel syndrome, allergies, and malabsorption. Boil all questionable water for at least twenty minutes at a rolling boil.

15

THE *BEYOND PRITIKIN* DIET MASTER STRATEGY

Now learn what and how great benefits a temperate diet will bring with it.
—HORACE

When you buy foods that are as near to nature as possible, you need not be concerned about deciphering food labels. It is only when foods are jarred, packaged, dehydrated, frozen, canned, pouched, or otherwise processed that we need to become alert to extra fat, salt, and sugar—not to mention over three thousand additives in the form of chemical preservatives, colorings, and flavorings.

A little primer will help to remedy the situation. There is a label pecking order that is easy to remember when doing your detective work on decoding. The first ingredient is the one found in the greatest quantity in the product, while the ingredient listed last is the one found in the least amount. Try to make sure that any questionable ingredient (such as processed fat, salt, sea salt, sugar, additives, or colorings) comes after the third item on the list.

Finding Fat

Fat, no matter what the label may read, is still considered fat and usually undesirable fat. Key words that can translate into trans, damaged, or excessive saturated fat include margarine, shortening, vegetable oil, mayonnaise, lard, suet, tallow, and mono-, di-, and triglycerides. Mineral oil is a nonnutritive substance that can flush fat-soluble vitamins out of the system, and should be avoided. A label that reads "100% vegetable oil" may not only be a heat-treated and therefore damaged oil, but it can be the cover for palm kernel or coconut oil—the most saturated oils of all.

Some oils that are not derived from food crops, such as cottonseed oil, are not subject to FDA regulations for pesticide safety. Cottonseed oil is often an ingredient in margarine—another reason to avoid it.

Sorting Out Salt

There is just as much misunderstanding about the importance of food sodium as there is about fats. Sodium is essential for good digestion, the acid/alkaline balance, and the lymph and blood fluid. Without enough sodium in the system, calcium can be precipitated and deposited in the joints, creating joint problems such as arthritis. Organic sodium is a potent neutralizer of excessive acidity. This is why cabbage juice, for example, which is naturally high in sodium, has such a healing effect on ulcers.

Unrefined Celtic Salt is a wonderful source of bio-organic sodium and valuable minerals. Other salts, such as common table salt and even most sea salts found in health food stores, are usually processed at extreme heat and devoid of the balancing accompanying minerals (magnesium, for example), leaving only sodium and chloride. The sodium in these products is ionized and crystallized. It hardens in the body, creating many of the problems we traditionally associate with too much salt, such as high blood pressure, kidney problems, and stiffness in the joints. Most of the salt found in seasonings, condiments, and packaged foods is refined, inorganic, and mineral deficient. By using a really natural, sun-dried, organic salt, digestion, assimilation, and elimination are improved.

Watch out for added inorganic sodium in the form of sodium combinations, brine, baking soda, and especially MSG (monosodium glutamate). Foods containing soy sauce or tamari should be shunned, as soy sauce packs a walloping 1,000 mg. of inorganic sodium per tablespoon. Although salt-reduced varieties contain only 500 mg. of sodium per tablespoon, you tend to use twice as much to attain the same flavor, and the problem of excess inorganic sodium remains.

The Yeast Problem: The Twentieth Century Epidemic

Many of my patients who eliminate soy sauce from their foods lose pounds of stored water weight. This fermented, wheat-containing product also contributes to yeast overgrowth and adds to systemic candidiasis—an increasing problem because of too much sugar, birth control pills, steroids, drugs, and unmonitored use of antibiotics.

Candida albicans has been aptly named the Twentieth Century Disease. Normally not a problem in a healthy body, the yeast overgrows in the intestines when the immune system is depressed. Antibiotics, whether taken directly for medical reasons or ingested indirectly through antibiotic-fed livestock, kill the beneficial intestinal microflora bacteria that normally control the *Candida.*

It is interesting to note that a *Candida*-control diet restricts sugar and high-carbohydrate foods, particularly those made from gluten-containing grains. Fruits and yeast-related foods such as mushrooms, cheeses, tomato sauces, soy sauce, and vinegar are also restricted or eliminated. All of these *Candida* considerations are built into the Master Menu Plan and dietary recommendations.

Sweet Surrender

With regard to hidden sugar, watch out for words ending in "ose," such as sucrose, dextrose, and lactose. Fructose (which is usually derived from corn, by the way) is the lowest sweetener on the Glycemic Index and so does not stimulate as high blood sugar levels as sucrose or maltose.

Where to Shop

Most of the staples for the *Beyond Pritikin* Diet can be purchased at your local supermarket or fruit and vegetable stand.* Extra virgin olive oil, for example, can be located in the specialty or gourmet section of the supermarket. Other *Beyond Pritikin* oils and nuts and seeds will more likely be found at your health food store, where whole grains, flours, thickeners, bulk grains, and cereals may also be located.

When shopping at your health food store, a word of caution is in order. The terms *natural* and *pure* have no real meaning in food advertising. You may think that there is a preselection of only "health" foods when in a natural foods store. However, most of the highly touted natural granola cereals, the pure and natural candy bars, and vegetarian frozen entrees usually contain as much fat as their supermarket equivalents. Nearly half the calories of a popular health food line of frozen entrees come from fat. And this company advertises its fare as "light and lean."

Health food stores stock high-fat products in the form of nut butters, raw-milk cheeses, full-fat yogurts, and

---

*Many of my patients clean their food in a special detoxifying bath that removes sprays, bacteria, fungus, parasites, and heavy metals. The formula is included on p. 149. For those who prefer to buy food from suppliers of organic foods who do not use animal drugs, pesticides, and sprays, see p. 151 for a list of organic food mail-order suppliers. This list is provided by *Safe Food* by Michael Jacobson (Living Planet Press, 1991.)

kefir. Salt adds up quickly in tamari, tempeh, and textured vegetable protein, while sugar masquerades in the form of blackstrap molasses, pure turbinado sugar, honey, rice syrup, and barley malt.

Before You Take a Bite

It has been said that it is not just the food that counts but what your body does with it. How true this is when you understand that we derive *no* value from foods that are not digested. Even Mark Twain knew that the average person "eats too much and chews too little!" Proper chewing to assure good digestion is of paramount importance. Although the main focus of the rest of this book is the 21-Day Master Menu Plan, which includes recipes, keep this nutritional fact in mind: this program will do you little good if your body can't absorb the nutrients you have so conscientiously prepared.

So, here is a most helpful hint to enhance digestion:

• Chew your food thoroughly—at least thirty times per bite, please.

Remember that ptyalin, the starch-digesting enzyme in saliva, is located in the mouth. The more you chew, the better your stomach and GI tract will behave.

Food Combinations

I have noticed over the years that with many patients, digestion and assimilation have improved when foods are combined in certain ways. While I don't endorse food combining per se, I can't help but note that intestinal discomfort such as gas, bloating, diarrhea, and constipation, as well as food allergies, may relate to incompatible food combinations. These observations have been built into the *Beyond Pritikin* Diet plan but bear repeating for personal menu planning and nutritional guidance. Try them out on yourself; your stomach may thank you forever.

These combinations appear to assist digestion:

• Protein and green vegetables. If you want to add starch, use rice, potato, millet, or corn. (Example: baked fish, green leafy salad, and brown rice.)

• Starch and vegetables. (Example: baked potato and steamed broccoli with carrots.)

• Melons eaten alone.

• Other fruits eaten at beginning of meal or between meals.

• Eggs seem to be neutral and can be enjoyed in most combinations. They complement beans, vegetables, and dairy products. They go well with the grain starches. (Example: omelets, quiche, and toast and eggs.)

These combinations can encourage digestive upsets:

• Flesh protein (fish, fowl, and beef) and gluten-rich grain starches (wheat, rye, oats, and barley). (Example: fillet of fish sandwich on a whole wheat bun.) The bran component from wheat and oats, however, does not contain gluten and can be used with flesh proteins.

• Vegetables and fruit eaten together. Save your fruit dessert for at least two hours after a vegetable meal. The exceptions to this rule are enzyme-rich papaya and pineapple, which are natural digestive aids and can be eaten with most foods.

• Milk and meat. (Example: a glass of milk with a roast beef dinner.)

• Water taken with meals before food is swallowed. While water is necessary for digestion, the saliva activity is weakened when water is used to wash down food. Extremely hot or cold water depresses gastric juices and acts as a shock to the system.

Stocking and Storing the Staples

Listed below are some basic foods with storage information that fit the criteria for *Beyond Pritikin* living. Brand names are used when generic product descriptions are not specific enough to assure high food quality and nutritive value suitable for the *Beyond Pritikin* Diet. For your convenience, several recommended brands are shown in parentheses but are not necessarily the only brands that meet quality standards.

The basic rule of thumb is to *buy right, then keep away from heat, air, and light!*

Oils

Unrefined safflower, sunflower, sesame, soy, corn, peanut, flaxseed, walnut, almond, hazelnut, canola (Super Canola, Arrowhead Mills, Erewhon, Norganic, Westbrae, Walnut Acres, Eden, Jaffe Brothers, Spectrum, Barlean's). Extra virgin and virgin olive oil (Siabica, Walnut Acres, Golden Eagle, Old Monk, Westbrae, Jaffe Brothers).

Most imported virgin oils from Spain, Greece, and Italy are acceptable. Remember that unprocessed oils contain sediment, are somewhat cloudy, and have a stronger taste, all signs of unrefined quality. The color of natural unrefined oils is related to the original source: olive oil is green, safflower oil is yellow, corn oil is orange, and soy oil is dark brown.

Storage Tips:
Refrigerate most oils in tightly capped bottles. Tinted glass or tin is the best storage protector. Olive oil can be kept in a cool, dark place. Buy

crude oil in small amounts and use it up within a short time after opening. Exposure to air and light can create rancidity.

Nuts and Seeds

Raw, unshelled almonds, filberts, pecans, walnuts; pumpkin, sunflower, poppy, caraway, flaxseed. Sesame seeds and sesame butter.

When selecting sesame seeds, choose a company that uses a mechanical hulling method rather than chemicals to dehull the seeds (International Protein Industries, Protein Aide, Arrowhead Mills, Westbrae). Nut butters other than sesame seed butter are not recommended because they can become rancid so easily. The oil in sesame seeds has great durability against rancidity.

Storage Tips:
Store nuts and seeds in the shell in the natural, unroasted state in a cool dry place. The refrigerator or freezer are good environments for nuts. Flaxseed especially must be ground right before cooking to avoid rancidity. Never use the whole flaxseed.

Mayonnaise

(Walnut Acres, Hain, Hollywood, Westbrae, Spectrum.)

Dairy

Nonfat milk, yogurt (Dannon, Nancy's, and Continental nonfat yogurt), and cottage cheese; sweet butter; grated Parmesan cheese occasionally; goat cheese, feta cheese, goat yogurt.

Dairy substitutes: fresh or powdered soymilk (Jolly Joan, Fearn, Energy

Foods); Rice Dream; tofu; soy cheese; almond cheese.

Storage Tips:
Keep milk and all milk products nearest the freezer section. Do not leave out more than two hours or cholesterol will oxidize.

Eggs: Fresh have the best flavor; use within one week of purchase.

Storage Tips:
To store separated eggs, pour cold water over the yolk and refrigerate up to four days. The egg white just needs to be covered with water.

Protein

Fish: All, especially the Omega-3 types such as salmon, mackerel, sardines, tuna, herring, trout, cod, flounder, butterfish, pilchard. Canned salmon, tuna, anchovies, mackerel. If packed in oil or salt, drain well under running water (Featherweight, Seasons, Lillie, Three Star).

Seafood: Shrimp, lobster, crab, scallops, calamari.

Poultry: White meat of skinned turkey and skinned chicken. Nitrate-free, uncured cooked turkey and chicken sausage (Health Valley, Harmony Farms).

Beef: Good or standard grades; flank, rump, round, chuck.

Buffalo ($3/8$ bison and $5/8$ bovine).

Lamb: Leg, loin, rib (avoid fatty shank and breast).

Veal: Shoulder, rib, loin (avoid fatty breast).

Venison

Tofu: In amounts comparable to fish, poultry, or lean meat.

Vegetables

All fresh in-season produce, when available. If fresh is not available, frozen is next best, followed by canned or jarred with no added salt. Water chestnuts, bamboo shoots, and artichoke hearts are readily available canned. Jarred fire-roasted red peppers are also on market shelves. Daikon radish, sunchokes (Jerusalem artichokes), and sprouted mixed beans make great nibbles and exotic salad additions. Low-sodium V-8 juice is good to keep on hand. See Vegetables listed on p. 226 under Food Equivalents for complete variety.

Fruits

Fresh, seasonally ripe, locally grown fruits are first choice when available and without mold. The next choice is frozen, and last is canned in natural unsweetened juices. See Fruits listed on p. 227 under Food Equivalents for complete variety.

Unsweetened fruit preserves, applebutter, and cranberry sauce conserve are also acceptable (Westbrae, Pure & Simple, Walnut Acres, Sorrell Ridge).

Fruit juices: Unsweetened apple, cherry, pineapple-coconut, pomegranate, papaya, cranberry, or cranberry sweetened with grape concentrate (Hansen, L&A, Walnut Acres, Shoosh, Wagners, Knudsen).

Grains   Unrefined whole grains such as whole pearl barley, bulgur, brown rice, buckwheat groats (kasha), corn meal, millet, steel-cut oats, rye, triticale, wild rice, whole wheat, kamut, spelt, quinoa, amaranth (Arrowhead Mills, Erewhon).

Storage Tips:
Store in air-tight containers for up to one month and then refrigerate. During the summer months, store in refrigerator after one week.

Cereals   Sugar-free, low-salt, no-preservative cereals hot and cold such as Wheatena, cream of rye, oat bran, cream of rice, 4- and 7-grain; barley flakes, oat flakes, corn flakes, soy grits, Nutri-Grain, shredded wheat, Grapenuts, Spicer's Hunger Crunchers. (Quaker, Kellogg's, Arrowhead Mills, Hadley's, Pure & Simple, Health Valley, New Morning, Erewhon, Barbara's).

Crackers   Scandinavian-style crisp breads, fiber crisps, rice snaps, rice tea cakes, rye crackers, whole wheat wafers, whole wheat matzo (Kavli, WasaBrod, AkMak, Fantastik Foods, Pacific Rice Products, Manischewitz).

Breads   Whole grain, free of chemicals and hydrogenated fats and processed oils. Pita, whole wheat, rye, spelt, English muffins, sprouted grain, Essene bread (Ezekial 4:9, Health Valley, Life

Stream, Food For Life, Cleopatra's, VitaSpelt). Rice cakes and corn tortillas.

Storage Tips:
Refrigerate or freeze to protect natural fats from becoming rancid with exposure to room-temperature air.

Pasta
Whole-wheat spaghetti, noodles, shells, and macaroni, corn pasta, spelt, kamut, cellophane rice and mung bean noodles, soba (buckwheat noodles) (Health Valley, de Boles, Malfun, Erewhon, Mrs. Leepers). Lupini pasta with 60% less gluten and four times more fiber than ordinary pasta is now available from IN-AG.

Flours
Soy, rice, barley, corn, whole wheat, potato, green split pea, lentil.

Storage Tips:
Store in cool, dry pantry for up to one month. After that, refrigerate. Corn meal must be refrigerated right away.

Baking powder
Aluminum-free such as Royal, Rumford, Price, Schillings. Low-sodium cereal-free by Cellu and Featherweight.

Thickeners
Arrowroot (also known as kuzu), quick tapioca, instant mashed potatoes, oat bran (Barbara's). Arrowroot is suggested because it adds extra calcium to foods and is easily digested.

Beans
Fresh, frozen, or well-drained canned. Garbanzo (chickpea), navy,

lima, pinto, black, split pea, lentil, soy, adzuki, black-eyed pea.

Storage Tips:
Store in air-tight glass containers away from light and heat.

Soups	Defatted chicken broth, lentil, split pea, minestrone, turkey rice, chicken vegetable (Health Valley, Walnut Acres, Pritikin, Hain's).
Flavor extracts	Pure almond, coconut, maple, anise, lemon, lime, orange, rum, vanilla (Bickford Flavors). Vanilla and almond together taste like butterscotch.
Herbs, spices, and condiments	Fresh or dried garlic, parsley, mustard, cayenne pepper, red pepper, black pepper, chili pepper, fennel, dill, horseradish, oregano, basil, sage, savory, rosemary, cumin, curry, ginger, tarragon, cinnamon, thyme, nutmeg, allspice, Chinese five-spice. Tabasco sauce, Worcestershire sauce, and Dijon mustard, Angostura bitters, capers.

Storage Tips:
Store dried herbs and spices in a cool place rather than above your stove where heat can affect them. The refrigerator or freezer tends to dry them out too much. A cool environment protects the volatile oils from warmth and moisture that change aromatic and pungent flavors.

Vinegars	Rice, wine, champagne, apple cider, raspberry, Balsamic, herb blends.

Salt	Celtic salt or solar-evaporated salt (De Souza).
Sweeteners	Raw, unheated honey, maple syrup, maple granules, date sugar; unsweetened fruit juices used sparingly for added flavors. Carob Dream (Choice Creations), Rice Dream, Stevia.

Wax Orchard's Classic Fudge Sweet is a fruit-sweetened version of the real thing . . . with no bad fats.

Avoid all artificial sweeteners, including aspartame. |
| Beverages | Herbal teas such as lemon grass, mint, pau d'areo, hibiscus, chamomile, rosehips, fennel, or taheebo (good for yeast problems); sparkling mineral waters.

Pure water is the best beverage of all. A good water filter that removes harmful bacteria, parasite cysts, and chemical pollutants is a necessity in this day and age. The Uni Key is the filter I personally now use and suggest to my patients because of the three-stage filtering method that blocks cryptosporidium. |
| Coffee substitutes | Dakopa (made from dahlia flower tubers), dandelion coffee, Pero, Postum, Pioneer, Bambu.

My clients say that Capri Mineral Whey (a dry natural food powder) is a pleasant coffee substitute that is truly delicious, with a mild caramel flavor. |
| Alcohol | For cooking and moderate drinking, use sulfite-free wines (Domaine de la |

Bousquette and Frey), vermouth, sherry, and Pernod. Vodka and sake (rice wine) for allergic individuals. Fruit liqueurs such as amaretto (almond), Grand Marnier (orange and cognac), Cointreau (orange), creme de menthe (mint), kirsch (cherry), and creme de cassis (black currant) enhance special desserts.

Gelatin   Agar-agar, a seaweed gelatin, replaces animal gelatin. Agar-agar provides added fiber and lubrication in the intestinal tract by absorbing moisture (Westbrae).

Balance Bars   Revolutionary meal or snack replacement that balances blood sugar. Flavors: Chocolate, Toasted Crunch, and Peanut. Call Uni Key.

Specialty Food and Water Filter Source

Uni Key Health Systems
P.O. Box 7168
Bozeman, MT 59771
(800) 888-4353

A Cleansing Formula

For the past 20 years, I have personally used and recommended this formula for elimination of food sprays, bacteria, fungus, parasites, and heavy metals without any report of adverse reaction. I first learned of the "Clorox bath" through Hazel Parcells, Ph.D., D.C., N.D. Military families stationed in Turkey, China, and Southeast Asia have also used it through the suggestion of the U.S. State Department. However, it is just as valuable and just as necessary here in America, where so many pesticides and chemical wastes are entering our food supply.

Clorox kills every known type of virus. If you're worried about the epidemic of salmonella in chickens, this treatment is the solution.

The following advantages have been reported over the years:

1. Allergic reaction is eliminated.
2. Fruits and vegetables taste "farm fresh" and keep twice as long.
3. Leafy greens retain their color and crispness.
4. Meats are tenderized with flavors enhanced.

If you are still concerned about pesticides and would rather not use Clorox, there is an alternative. A product called Fit Produce Rinse is now on the market and is said to remove almost 90 percent of chemicals and wax on most fruits and vegetables. The Fit Produce Rinse is approved by *Good Housekeeping* and consists of just baking soda and citric acid. You can call 1-800-4FIT-FIT for more information.

The Formula

1. Use ½ teaspoon Clorox to 1 gallon of water, obtained from the usual source. Only the Clorox brand will work, so do not substitute any other product.

2. Place the foods to be treated into the bath according to the chart below. Make a separate bath for each group.

3. Remove foods from the Clorox bath and place in clear water for ten minutes. Dry all foods thoroughly, and store.

Food Group	Treatment Time
Vegetables	
Leafy vegetables	15 minutes
Root vegetables, thick-skinned or fibrous vegetables	30 minutes
Fruits	
Thin-skinned berries, peaches, apricots, plums	15 minutes

Thick-skinned fruits such as apples, citrus, and bananas	30 minutes
Chicken, fish, meats, eggs	20 minutes

Note: Meats can be thawed in a Clorox bath. The timing is about 20 minutes for a weight of 2 to 5 pounds. Frozen turkey or chicken should remain in the Clorox bath until thawed. Ground meats, of course, cannot be Cloroxed.

Mail Order Suppliers of Organic Food

The following growers and distributors can ship their products directly, usually via UPS, and do not require a minimum order unless otherwise noted. Write or call them for complete product listings.

All of the following suppliers have their certification method indicated with one of three letters: "C" indicates that all products listed have been certified organic by an independent certifying organization or agency. "S" means that the suppliers have established their own organic standards and are considered self-certified. "V" signifies that certification varies and products are labeled accordingly.

ARIZONA

Arjoy Acres
HCR Box 1410
Payson, AZ 85541
(602) 474-1224
Garlic, dried beans and peas. (S)

ARKANSAS

Dharma Farma
Star Route Box 140
Osage, AR 72638
(501) 553-2550
Apples, pears. (C)

Eagle Agricultural
Products

2223 N. College
Fayetteville, AR 72703
(501) 442-6792
Fresh and dried produce, beans, grains, pasta, flour. (V)

Good Earth Association
202 E. Church St.
Pocahontas, AR 72455
(501) 892-9545
(501) 892-8329
Corn, beans, seed crops. (S)

Mountain Ark Trading
Company

120 South East Ave.
Fayetteville, AR 72701
AR: (501) 442-7191
US: 1-800-643-8909
Grains, beans, seeds, wide
selection of products. (V)

CALIFORNIA

Ahler's Organic Date
Garden
P.O. Box 726
Mecca, CA 92254-0726
(619) 396-2337
Dates, date products. (S)

Blue Heron Farm
P.O. Box 68
Rumsey, CA 95679
(916) 796-3799
Almonds, walnuts,
oranges. (C)
Minimum order varies.

Covalda Date Co.
P.O. Box 908
Coachella, CA 92236
(619) 398-3441
Dates, dried fruits and
nuts. (S)

Capay Fruits and
Vegetables
23800 State Hwy. 16
Capay, CA 95607
(916) 796-4111
Dried tomatoes, peaches,
herbs. (C)

Ecology Sound Farms
42126 Road 168
Orosi, CA 93647
(209) 528-3816
(209) 528-2276
Oranges, plums, Asian pears,
kiwi fruit, persimmons. (C)

Minimum order 8-40 lbs.
depending on item.

Frey Vineyards
14000 Tomki Road
Redwood Valley, CA
95470
(707) 485-5177
Wine. (C)
Minimum order ½ case.

Gold Mine Natural Food
Co.
1947 30th Street
San Diego, CA 92102
1-800-475-FOOD
Brown rices, beans, mac-
robiotic items, wide variety of goods. (V)

Gravelly Ridge Farms
Star Route 16
Elk Creek, CA 95939
(916) 963-3216
Produce, grains. (C)

Great Date in the
Morning
P.O. Box 31
Coachella, CA 92236
(619) 398-6171
Dates. (C)

Green Knoll Farm
P.O. Box 434
Gridley, CA 95948
(916) 846-3431
Kiwifruit. (C)
Minimum order 7.5 lbs.

Jaffe Brothers
P.O. Box 636
Valley Center, CA 92082-
0636
(619) 749-1133
Dried fruit, nuts, grains,
beans, assorted goods. (S)

Living Tree Centre
P.O. Box 10082
Berkeley, CA 94709
(415) 420-1440
Almonds, almond butter,
pistachios, apple trees. (C)

Lundberg Family Farm
P.O. Box 369
Richvale, CA 95974-0369
(916) 882-4551
Rice and rice products.
(C)

Mendocino Sea
Vegetable Co.
P.O. Box 372
Navarro, CA 95463
(707) 895-3741
Wildcrafted sea vegetables
(harvested seaweed). (S)

Natural Gardening
Company
217 San Anselmo Ave.
San Anselmo, CA 94960
(415) 456-5060
Vegetable seedlings. (C)
Minimum order 1 flat.

Old Mill Farm School of
Country Living
P.O. Box 463
Mendocino, CA 95460
(707) 937-0244
Lamb, goat cheese, pro-
duce. (C)
Minimum order $50.

Steven Pavich and Sons
Rt. 2, Box 291
Delano, CA 93215
(805) 725-1046
Grapes. (C)

Sleepy Hollow Farm
44001 Dunlap Road
Miramonte, CA 93641

(209) 336-2444
Apples, cooking herbs.
(C)
Minimum order 1 box.

Soghomonian Farms
8624 S. Chestnut
Fresno, CA 93725
(209) 834-2772
Grapes in season, raisins.
(C)

Timber Crest Farms
4791 Dry Creek Road
Healdsburg, CA 95448
(707) 433-8251
Wide variety of dried
fruits and nuts. (S)

Weiss' Kiwifruit
594 Paseo Companeros
Chico, CA 95928
(916) 343-2354
Kiwifruit. (C)
Minimum order 2½ lbs.

COLORADO

Malachite Small Farm
School
ASR Box 21, Pass Creek
Road
Gardner, CO 81040
(719) 746-2412
Honey, quinoa, beef. (S)

Wilton's Organic
Potatoes
Box 28
Aspen, CO 81612
(303) 925-3433
Potatoes. (C)
Minimum order 5 lbs.

CONNECTICUT

Butterbrooke Farm
78 Barry Road

Oxford, CT 06483
(203) 888-2000
Vegetable seeds. (C)

FLORIDA

Sprout Delights
13090 N.W. 7th Ave.
Miami, FL 33168-2702
(305) 687-5880
1-800-334-2253
Full line of bakery items.
(S)

Starr Organic Produce
P.O. Box 561502
Miami, FL 33256-1502
(305) 262-1242
Wide variety of fruit. (S)
Minimum order 20 lbs.

HAWAII

Hawaiian Exotic
Fruit Co.
Box 1729
Pahoa, HI 96778
(808) 965-7154
Dried pineapples,
bananas, papaya, fresh
ginger root, turmeric. (S)
Minimum order 10 lbs.

IDAHO

Ronnigers Seed Potatoes
Star Route
Moyie Springs, ID 83845
(208) 267-7938
Vegetables. (S)
Minimum order $10.

ILLINOIS

Green Earth Natural
Foods
2545 Prairie Avenue
Evanston, IL 60201

1-800-322-3662
(708) 864-8949
Fresh produce, meats,
wide variety of items. (V)

Nu-World Amaranth
P.O. Box 2202
Naperville, IL 60540
(708) 369-6819
Amaranth flour, cereal,
whole grain. (C)

IOWA

Frontier Cooperative
Herbs
P.O. Box 299
Norway, IA 52318
1-800-365-4372
(319) 227-7991
Herbs, spices, teas. (V)

Nature's Korner
R2 Box 302
Iowa Falls, IA 50126
(515) 648-9568
Large selection of gro-
ceries, specializes in
breads. (S)

Paul's Grains
2475-B 340 St.
Laurel, IA 50141
(515) 476-3373
Whole grains and grain
products, beef, lamb,
chicken, turkey. (S)

KENTUCKY

Gracious Living Farm
General Delivery
Insko, KY 41443
Vegetables. (S)

Prosperity Farms
550 Gardener Road
Magnolia, KY 42757

(502) 528-2422
Condiments, pesto, pick-
les, salsa, etc. (S)
Minimum order varies.

MAINE

Crossroad Farms
Box 3230
Jonesport, ME 04649
(207) 497-2641
Root crops, squash, cab-
bage, apples. (C)
Minimum order $25.

Fiddler's Green Farm
R.R. 1, Box 656
Belfast, ME 04915
(207) 338-3568
Whole grain mixes, cof-
fee, syrup, and jam. (V)

Johnny's Selected Seeds
Foss Hill Road
Albion, ME 04910
(207) 437-4301
Vegetable, herb, and farm
seeds. (S)

Maine Coast Sea
Vegetables
Shore Road
Franklin, ME 04634
(207) 565-2907
Sea chips, kelp, dulse,
nori. (S)

Simply Pure Food
RFD #3, Box 99
Bangor, ME 04401
(207) 848-7371
Strained and diced baby
foods, baby cereals. (C)

Wood Prairie Farm
RFD 1 Box 164S
Bridgewater, ME 04735
(207) 429-9765

Maple syrup, oats and oat
products, various vegeta-
bles. (C)

MARYLAND

Macrobiotic Mall
18779-C N. Frederick
Ave.
Gaithersburg, MD 20879
(301) 963-9235
Grains, legumes, packaged
foods, macrobiotic items.
(C)

Organic Foods Express
11003 Emack Road
Beltsville, MD 20705
(301) 816-4944
Produce, grains, beans,
coffee, assorted goods. (V)

MASSACHUSETTS

Baldwin Hill Bakery
Baldwin Hill Road
Phillipston, MA 01331
(508) 249-4691
Sourdough bread. (C)
Minimum order 6 loaves.

Cooks' Maple Products
Bashan Hill Road
Worthington, MA 01098
(413) 238-5827
Maple syrup. (S)

Greek Gourmet, Ltd.
5 Pond Park Road
Hingham, MA 02043
(617) 749-1866
Extra virgin olive oil,
olives. (S)
Minimum order 1 case.

MICHIGAN

Country Life Natural
Foods

109th Ave.
Pullman, MI 49450
(616) 236-5011
Bulk natural foods. (V)

Eugene and Joan Saintz
2225 63rd
Fennville, MI 49408
(616) 561-2761
Fresh produce in season.
(S)

Todd Gulich
Nature's Market Whole
Foods
139 West Auburn
Rochester Hill, MI 48307
(313) 852-9327
Produce, meats, grains,
herbs, and other foods.
(V)

MINNESOTA

Diamond K Enterprises
R.R. 1 Box 30A
St. Charles, MN 55972
(507) 932-4308; 932-
5433
Grains and grain prod-
ucts, nuts, dried fruits.
(C)

French Meadow Bakery
2610 Lyndale Ave., So.
Minneapolis, MN 55408
(612) 870-4740
Many sourdough breads.
(C)
Minimum order $20.

Living Farms
Box 50
Tracy, MN 56175
US: 1-800-533-5320
MN: 1-800-622-5235

Grains, sprouting seeds.
(V)

Mill City Sourdough
Bakery
2070 Grand Ave.
St. Paul, MN 55105
(612) 699-4784
1-800-87-DOUGH
Sourdough breads. (C)
Minimum order 6 loaves.

Natural Way Mills, Inc.
Rt. 2, Box 37
Middle River, MN 56737
(218) 222-3677
Whole grains, flours, cere-
als, other products. (C)

MONTANA

The Good Food Store
920 Kensington
Missoula, MT 59801
(406) 728-5823
Beans, grains, dried fruits
and vegetables, cereals,
coffee and tea, pasta,
seeds, spices. (V)
Minimum order $25.

NEBRASKA

Do-R-Dye Organic Mill
Box 50, Route 1
Rosalie, NE 68055
(402) 863-2248
Oats, wheat, rye, corn
products. (S)
Minimum order $5.

M and M Distributing
RR 2, Box 61-A
Oshkosh, NE 69154
(308) 772-3664
Whole grain armaranth.
(S)
Minimum order 25 lbs.

Stapelman Meats
Rt. 2, Box 6A
Belden, NE 68717
(402) 985-2470
Beef, pork. (S)

NEW HAMPSHIRE

Water Wheel Sugar
House
Rt. 2
Jefferson, NH 03583
(603) 586-4479
Maple syrup. (S)

NEW JERSEY

Simply Delicious
243 A N. Hook Rd.,
Box 124
Pennsville, NJ 08070
(609) 678-4488
Wide variety of items. (V)

NEW MEXICO

Blue Corn Trading
Company
Box 951
Taos Pueblo, NM 87571
(505) 758-4803
Blue corn flour, herbs. (S)

NEW YORK

Bread Alone
Rt. 28
Boiceville, NY 12412
(914) 657-3328
Wheat, rye and sour-
dough breads. (C)
Minimum order 12
loaves.

Community Mill and
Bean
267 Rt. 89 S
Savannah, NY 13146

(315) 365-2664
Flour, mixes, beans,
grains, cereals. (C)
Minimum order $10.

Deer Valley Farm
R.D. 1
Guilford, NY 13780
(607) 764-8556
Meats, produce, grains,
baked goods, wide variety
of products. (V)
Minimum order $10.

Four Chimneys Farm
Winery
RD #1, Hall Road
Himrod, NY 14842
(607) 243-7502
Wine, grape juice, wine
vinegar. (C)
Minimum order for juice
1 case.

Gaeta Imports Inc.
141 John St.
Babylon, NY 11702-2903
(516) 661-2681
1-800-669-2681
Capers, porcini, olives,
and olive oil. (V)

NORTH CAROLINA

American Forest Foods
Corp.
Rt. 5, Box 84E
Henderson, NC 27536
(919) 438-2674
Shiitake and oyster mush-
rooms, mixes, spices. (C)
Minimum order 10 packs.

OHIO

Earth's Best
Hand in Hand Catalogue
9180 LeSaint Dr.

Fairfield, OH 45014
1-800-543-4343
Baby food: purees, cereals,
juices. (C)
Minimum order 12 jars.

OREGON

Dement Creek Farms
Box 155
Broadbent, OR 97414
(503) 572-5564
Beans, grains, vegetables,
herbs. (C)

Herb Pharm
20260 Williams Hwy.
Williams, OR 97544
(503) 846-6262
Herbs, herbal extracts,
teas. (C)
Minimum order $25.

Mountain Springs
P.O. Box 861
Prineville, OR 97754
1-800-542-2303
Canned and smoked rain-
bow trout. (S)

River Bend Organic Farm
and Country Store
2363 Tucker Road
Hood River, OR 97031
(503) 386-8766
Fresh fruit, jams, syrup. (C)

PENNSYLVANIA

Dutch Country Gardens
Box 1122 Road #1
Tamaqua, PA 18252
(717) 668-0441
Potatoes, carrots. (S)
Minimum order $25.

Garden Spot Distributors
438 White Oak Road

New Holland, PA 17557
(717) 354-4936
Wide variety of dried and
packaged goods. (V)

Genesee Natural Foods
R.D. 2, Box 105
Genesee, PA 16923
(814) 228-3200
(814) 228-3205
Beans, grains, flours,
honey, pasta, cereals,
dried fruit. (V)
Minimum order $20.

Krystal Wharf Farms
RD 2, Box 2112
Mansfield, PA 16933
(717) 549-8194
Grains, beans, nuts, dried
fruit, seeds, fresh produce,
and other products.
(C)(S)

Rising Sun Distributors
P.O. Box 627
Milesburg, PA 16853
(814) 355-9850
Produce, dried fruit, nuts,
beans, grains, other items.
(V)

Walnut Acres
Walnut Acres Road
Penns Creek, PA 17862
(717) 837-0601
Full line of cereals, flours,
grains, baked goods,
soups, vegetables, other
items. (S)

PUERTO RICO

Finca del Seto Cafe
P.O. Box 30
Jayuya, PR 00664-0030

Whole and ground coffee. (S)

TEXAS

Arrowhead Mills
Box 2059
Hereford, TX 79045
(806) 364-0730
A wide variety of grains
and grocery items. (C)

Stanley Jacobson
1505 Doherty
Mission, TX 78572
(512) 585-1712
Grapefruit and oranges.
(C)
Minimum order ¼ bushel.

Lee's Organic Foods
Box 111
Wellington, TX 79095
(806) 447-5445
Fruit jerkies. (C)
Minimum order $25.

VERMONT

Gourmet Produce Co.
RR 3, Box 348
Chester, VT 05143
(802) 875-3820
Sunflower and radish
sprouts, wheatgrass and
wheatgrass juice. (C)

Hill and Dale Farms
Rt. 2, Box 1260
West Hill-Daniel Davis
Road
Putney, VT 05346
(802) 387-5817
Apples, vinegar. (S)
Minimum order 1 flat
(24 apples.)

Northeast Kingdom
Organic
RR1, Box 608
Hardwick, VT 05843
(802) 472-5710
(802) 472-6019
Root-cellar vegetables,
dried beans and herbs,
canned goods. (C)

Teago Hill Farm
Barber Hill Road
Pomfret, VT 05067
(802) 457-3507
Maple syrup. (S)

VIRGINIA

Golden Acres Orchard
Rt. 2, Box 2450
Front Royal, VA 22630
(703) 636-9611
Apples in season, cider
vinegar, juice. (S)

Golden Angels Apiary
P.O. Box 2
Singers Glen, VA 22850
(703) 833-5104
Five types of honey. (S)

Natural Beef Farms
4399-A Henninger Court
Chantilly, VA 22021
(703) 631-0881
Frozen meats, produce,
bread, wide variety of
items. (C)

WASHINGTON

Cascadian Farm
P.O. Box 568
Concrete, WA 98237
(206) 853-8175
Fruit conserves, dill pick-
les. (C)

Homestead Organic
Produce
2002 Road 7 NW
Quincy, WA 98848
(509) 787-2248
Onions, garlic, apples. (C)
Minimum order varies.

Sunny Pine Farm
Rte. 2, Box 280
Twisp, WA 98856
(509) 997-4811
Garlic and garlic prod-
ucts. (C)

WEST VIRGINIA

Brier Run Farm
Rt. 1, Box 73
Birch River, WV 26610
(304) 649-2975
Goat cheeses (Chèvre).
(C)
Minimum order $25.

Hardscrabble Enterprises,
Inc.
Route 6, Box 42
Cherry Grove, WV 26804
(304) 358-2921; (202)
332-0232
Dried shiitake mush-
rooms. (S)
Minimum order 1 box
(1½ lbs.).

WISCONSIN

Joel Afdahl
Route, 1 Box 1580
Hammond, WI 54015
(715) 796-5395
Maple syrup. (S)

Nokomis Farm
3293 Main Street
East Troy, WI 53120
(414) 642-9665
Grains, breads, beef, pork.
(C)

Special Salad Dressings

There are a number of acceptable salad dressings in
both supermarkets and health food stores. Look for
dressings made by Spectrum and Blanchard &
Blanchard.

A Note About Irradiated Food

There is a controversy about the safety of eating irradiated food, a process that extends shelf life by using ioniz-
ing radiation. Aside from the questionable safety factor,
I personally feel that since there are so many conditions

Source: Jacobson, Michael. *Safe Food*. (Venice, CA, and Washington, D.C. Living
Planet Press, 1991.)

in our society today that devitalize and contaminate food, I am not in favor of adding another one. If you want further information on this topic contact: Food and Water, Inc., Depot Hill Road, R.R. 1, Box 114, Marshfield, VT 05658 (802) 426-3700.

16

ABOUT THE DIET: QUESTIONS AND ANSWERS

The food you eat today, walks around tomorrow.
—Dr. Hazel Parcells

Q. Is fruit a major part of the food plan as it is in recent popular diets?

A. No.

A *maximum* of three fruit portions per day is the most you should consume. A portion equals one-half grapefruit, for example, or ten cherries, one medium peach, one small orange, two medium prunes, or twelve grapes. (See Food Equivalents on p. 224 for a complete list.) Note that on the *Beyond Pritikin* Diet fruits are consumed first thing at breakfast or as between-meal snacks. Some research indicates that when fruit is eaten after meals or with the meal, the fructose content can be more easily converted to fat.

I have reviewed too many diet histories and coordinating blood values not to notice that people who eat large amounts of fruit have high triglyceride values and a disturbed calcium balance. With more medical attention focused on preventing osteoporosis, a degenerative bone disease that affects 15 to 20 million postmenopausal American women, it makes good nutritional sense to cut out calcium-lowering sugar and limit even natural sugar sources from excess fruit, for example, and even fruit juice.

In addition to unbalancing mineral ratios in the body, excessive sugar can also block essential fat conversion into prostaglandins. Essential fat itself helps to maintain calcium levels in the blood by delivering it to the soft tissues.

Vegetarians, I have often observed, will eat an entire meal of only fruit. They should concentrate instead on more protein-rich beans and whole grains for balanced nourishment.

The body does not differentiate between the sources of sugar. Too much of a sweet thing—whether refined or natural—can result in problems, so all sweets, *including fruit*, should be monitored. Excessive sugar consumption is often connected with dental cavities, diabetes, depression, hypoglycemia, and hyperactivity. It may also lower resistance to viruses and colds, or depress immune system response.

Q. I am on a low-salt diet. Is the *Beyond Pritikin* Diet sodium-restricted?
A. Yes.
The *Beyond Pritikin* Master Plan is also a controlled sodium diet containing less than 1500 mg. of sodium per day. The use of added salt is optional in all of the recipes; however, even with the added salt, the total daily amount does not exceed 1500 mg. If you do choose to omit the salt, use a suitable salt substitute to preserve flavor. Excessive inorganic sodium consumption may contribute to high blood pressure and water retention. Both the preferred salt and sweetening choices have been listed under "Stocking and Storing the Staples" (p. 141).

Q. Are dairy products recommended?
A. Certain dairy products are recommended.
Homogenized whole or low-fat milk products are avoided because of the presence of the destructive en-

zyme xanthine oxidase (XO). XO has been associated with artery damage, and is easily absorbed by the body in the dispersed milkfat. Low-fat milk (2 percent) is not recommended either, because it derives over 30 percent of its calories from homogenized milkfat. Nonfat milk, cheese, and yogurt are permitted because technically they contain no fat and are a source of calcium. If you suspect a sensitivity to dairy products or experience sinus problems, I suggest you eliminate all dairy items from the diet. One of the insidious effects of food sensitivity is weight gain due to retention of fluid (edema) because of an inflammatory reaction in the tissues.

Goat milk, cheese, and yogurt are recommended as the ideal dairy sources because they are not homogenized. They are also better tolerated by many individuals, hence less allergenic, than milk products from cows. There are many first-rate goat cheeses now available, since goat cheese production in the United States has increased in the last few years.

Yogurt cheese is a deliciously simple snack. Nutmeg, cinnamon, cardamom, or vanilla extract can add an extra dash of flavor. You will need to make the yogurt cheese one day ahead. The recipe calls for just 1 cup (one 8-ounce container) of nonfat yogurt. Pour the yogurt into a cheesecloth-lined colander that is set over a bowl. Cover and refrigerate for 24 hours. You will have ½ cup of yogurt cheese in a day.

Q. What about coffee?
A. No.

Coffee is also not recommended because it contains caffeine, a detrimental nerve stimulant, and irritating volatile oils. Caffeine stimulates the adrenal glands, causing adrenaline to be released into the bloodstream. Adrenaline activates our fight-or-flight response, increasing our heart rate, blood pressure, and blood sugar. When this initial rush wears off, blood sugar drops to lower levels than before the coffee and leaves the adrenal glands in a depleted state. And then it's time for another cup of coffee.

When sugar is added, the problem is intensified because refined sugars have the same stressful effect on the adrenal glands. Frequent use of coffee exhausts the adrenal glands and probably is the most central factor in low blood sugar in coffee drinkers. This also applies to chocolate, which contains caffeine and a related substance, theobromine.

Coffee may also irritate sensitive intestinal membranes. It interferes with the absorption of minerals, especially magnesium and iron. It depletes vitamins B and C, and alters the balance of neurotransmitters in the brain. University studies have shown that drinking more than two cups of coffee per day also elevates cholesterol levels.

Decaffeinated coffee also has detrimental effects on the body. Some decaffeination processes leave chemical residues such as methylene chloride, which is toxic to the liver and causes cancer in laboratory animals. Water extraction or Swiss process decaffeination is safer; however, most of the negative effects of coffee remain. Whether decaffeinated or not, imported coffees contain insecticide residues that are prohibited in this country.

Q. What about alcohol?
A. Yes.
Alcohol can be used in cooking but not consumed as a beverage. Moderate to heavy alcohol consumption blocks prostaglandin production. Wine and sherry are used in the recipes because, when used for cooking, most of the alcohol is burned off while the flavor remains. Alcohol burn-off takes about half an hour when food is simmering in soups and stews. It burns off in three minutes when used to sauté.

While there is evidence that it may raise beneficial HDL cholesterol levels, taken straight and in excessive amounts (more than a couple of beers, two small glasses of wine, or two mixed drinks), alcohol can have detrimental effects on the body. It interferes with the utilization of the essential fatty acids; it can prematurely age the skin, causing drying, wrinkling, and loss of elasticity. Other medical problems of excessive alcohol use include cirrhosis of the liver (fatty liver), malnutrition (empty calories, reduced stomach-acid secretion, altered digestive system), depression, and blood sugar instability.

Grain-sensitive individuals may react badly to alcoholic beverages derived from grains such as wheat, rye, corn, barley, and hops. If you suspect that you are one of these individuals, use vodka (from potatoes) or sake (rice wine). The sulfite preservative used in most wines can also have ill effects on asthmatic, allergic, and sensitive individuals.

Some alcoholism is genetically based. Certain races (such as the American Indians) or families with a history of alcoholism have a defective liver enzyme that metabolizes alcohol. Such people experience irritation of the nervous system and intense cravings for more alcohol. These individuals should completely avoid all alcohol.

Q. Are soft drinks allowed?
A. No.

Soft drinks are not recommended because they contain refined sugar or sugar substitutes such as aspartame (NutraSweet) or saccharine. Refined sugar depletes the body of B vitamins and unbalances calcium/phosphorus ratios.

Sugar substitutes such as saccharine have been known to cause liver damage to test animals at high doses. Aspartame, the most recently developed sugar substitute, is composed of the two amino acids phenylalanine and aspartic acid, and wood alcohol (methanol). It has been implicated in a wide range of complaints, including seizures, high blood pressure, visual impairment, dizziness, headaches, and dry eye syndrome.

Q. Do you suggest extra vitamins and minerals?
A. Yes.

The inclusion of a multivitamin and mineral supplement

that contains the necessary co-factors for essential fat conversion is a dietary necessity for several reasons:

1. It is included because without the necessary vitamins—such as niacin, B-6, C, zinc, and magnesium—GLA and EPA cannot convert into the protective prostaglandins. Weight loss also may be inhibited. I suggest using a supplement to assure the inclusion of the essential vitamins and minerals because food sources for these nutrients may be unreliable due to topsoil depletion (zinc), food processing (depletes B-6 and magnesium), and storage time (vitamin C) before the food gets to your table.

2. The nutrient tables from agricultural handbooks, or such an esteemed nutritional reference as Bowes and Church's *Food Values of Portions Commonly Used,* are not accurate reflections of how much nutrition is in our foods when we eat them. The vitamin and mineral levels are determined right after food has been harvested. These levels do not reflect the decrease in value by the canning process, in which up to 80 percent of vitamins are lost, or by freezing, in which up to 45 percent of vitamins are lost.

3. Then there is environmental pollution that creates a vitamin and mineral deficit. Each year we are exposed to more than 200,000 tons of air pollutants per person, and ingest 5 pounds of food additives and 120 pounds of sugar. In addition, there is the massive variety of pesticides and industrial wastes in both water and food. These substances deplete nutrients from our bodies in the process of detoxifying and eliminating them. Pollution necessitates more vitamins A, C, and E. Smoking destroys 25 mg. of vitamin C *per cigarette.* Chlorinated drinking water eats up more vitamin E, and glaring fluorescent office lights strain the body's supply of vitamin A.

4. Medications such as aspirin, cold remedies, and tranquilizers cancel out nutrients. Birth control pills create a need for additional B-6 and B-12, as well as folic acid. Alcohol eliminates the B vitamins, and a lack of thi-

amin (vitamin B-1) is linked to marginal malnutrition similar to beriberi among today's adolescents, who eat excessive amounts of junk food.

5. Psychological stress can require increased supplementation of one or more nutrients. The *American Physician Family Journal* advises that "all recent surveys indicate that Americans lack calcium, iron, magnesium, B-6, and zinc"—three of the five necessities for good-fat utilization.

Consult your nutritionally oriented doctor for more specific guidance beyond the multiple vitamin/mineral supplement suggested here. (I recommend Female Formula or Male Formula—see page 92.) Remember that vitamins in mega amounts act like drugs on the body. The same pharmacological effects can be experienced with herbs, because herbs are the original "medicants" from which modern day drugs are derived. Digitalis comes from foxglove, and belladonna from the herb by the same name. Valium is a derivative of the valerian root, and aspirin has its roots in willow bark. So be careful when using any of these without professional guidance.

Q. Why are portions given for fruit and protein if weight loss is not the concern?

A. In order to get the most out of the *Beyond Pritikin* Diet, you need to understand the chemistry behind it. The specific amounts (i.e., 4 ounces or ½ cup) of fruit and protein must be followed exactly as shown because of their connection with mineral balance that affects the prostaglandins. Too much fruit can create mineral loss by upsetting the calcium/phosphorus ratio, which in turn depletes other available minerals that are needed as co-factors in prostaglandin metabolism. Similarly, excess protein can drain the body's mineral reserves, depleting the available minerals used for prostaglandins.

Q. What should be limited for weight loss?

A. If you are overweight or inactive, and have not been using unrefined oils or supplementing with GLA directly, you are not adequately metabolizing high-calorie foods. This is why daily amounts of cereals, breads, starchy vegetables, and beans are also given— but in parentheses, because not everybody needs to lose weight. After the initial three-week phase, portions given in the parentheses can be increased in ½ cup increments until you can eat all you want without gaining weight.

Remember that when your fat burner is normalized and nutritionally sustained with the unrefined vegetable oils and/or preformed GLA supplements, appetite will naturally decrease and you will be satisfied with smaller portions. You will not have to resort to willpower or tedious calorie counting to prevent overeating.

Balanced metabolism is the goal. The elimination of sugar, trans fats, and alcohol will not only allow the oils to help you metabolize greater calories, it will prevent dips in blood sugar levels that cause you to overeat.

Q. How does butter figure into the diet?

A. The use of additional butter to the diet, other than the trace amounts contained in certain recipes in the menu, is not recommended until weight loss has been stabilized. Although butter can theoretically be designated a healthy fat when eaten in moderation, it does not contain enough of the cis-linoleic fatty acid to convert to fat-burning GLA and therefore cannot assist in initial weight loss. Once weight loss is maintained, butter can be added in the amounts of 1 to 2 teaspoons per meal as long as the unrefined oils are still included in equal amounts.

The *Beyond Pritikin* Diet Master Menu Plan is designed to be safe for everybody in every aspect. Variety is a key feature of the plan, so you will note that the same foods are not repeated every day. Variety eating thereby ensures the consumption of a wide range of vegetables, fruits, protein, and complex carbohydrates. This gives the body maximum exposure to all fifty nutrients from food sources. Mother Nature has blessed us with more than sixty varieties of vegetables and more than twenty kinds of fruits and beans. When meals are planned according to nutritional value and appeal, color inevitably comes into play. Colorful meals provide particular nutritional assistance. In foods colored orange and yellow, vitamin A is highlighted; red and blue foods provide iron-rich nutrition, while green foods give us magnesium.

From the overweight to the allergic to the high-risk cardiovascular patient to the individual wanting to improve his or her immune system—everyone can enjoy the fruits of the *Beyond Pritikin* system.

The Eleven-Point Prescription

The Eleven-Point Prescription is a summary of the *Beyond Pritikin* approach. These eleven practical guidelines are designed for sustained weight loss and long-term health.

1. Eliminate all sources of damaged fats, such as commercial vegetable oils, hydrogenated oil products (margarine and vegetable shortening), and all products containing them (read the labels). Use only purified, unrefined, expeller-pressed, raw or virgin oils.

2. Avoid dried, cured, and aged animal foods (powdered milk, dried eggs, and aged cheese such as Parmesan).

3. Eliminate whole or low-fat homogenized cow's milk, yogurt, and cheese. Nonfat dairy products, in which there is no fat content, are permitted. Goat's milk, yogurt, and cheese are acceptable.

4. At fast food restaurants, avoid hot dogs, hamburgers, bacon, chicken, french fries and onion rings, fish, mayonnaise, salad dressings, sauces, and sodas. It's okay to have a salad if you bring your own essential-fat dressing.

5. Consume at least three fish meals per week (favor salmon, mackerel, sardines, tuna, trout, cod, crab, and shrimp).

6. Include two tablespoons of essential fat every day in salad dressings and cooking. (Use only olive, canola, or peanut oil when cooking.)

7. Include up to but not more than three whole, portion-controlled fruits per day.

8. Eat high-fiber oats, beans, vegetables, and fruits.

9. Use onion, garlic, lemon, herbs, flavor extracts, and alcohol in cooking to season food. To prevent yeast problems, limit mustards, vinegars, tomato sauces, and soy sauce.

10. Drink at least eight glasses of water per day from sources such as spring, mineral, or filtered. Herbal tea or coffee substitutes should be made from these waters.

11. Balance meals with a combination of protein, carbohydrates, and the right fats. Try to choose carbohydrates that are lower on the Glycemic Index for everyday consumption.

17

THE TWO-WEEK FAT FLUSH

*The human body has one ability not
possessed by any machine—
the ability to repair itself.*
—George E. Kriley, Jr., M.D.

The Two-Week Fat Flush is a quick way to cleanse the accumulated bad fats in the tissues and liver. It also prevents new fats, in the form of triglycerides, from forming and reestablishes a beneficial fat ratio in the brown fat tissues for continued weight stabilization, fat-burning stimulation, and appetite control.

Some people lose up to 10 inches at the waist, buttocks, and thighs, whereas they may lose only 5 pounds on the scale. This two-week plan flushes out fat that normal diets don't. On this companion program to the *Beyond Pritikin* Diet Master Strategy, you will lose weight and begin to metabolize the toxic water and fat accumulation in your body.

If you are doing the program mainly for weight loss, weigh yourself only once a week. People do not lose weight at the same rate and you can get discouraged if you hit a plateau. You can completely redistribute your weight on this program without a dramatic loss on the scale.

Give Your Liver a Vacation

The *fat flush* gives the liver a well-deserved vacation from its many functions. The liver synthesizes and normalizes blood protein, stores glycogen, normalizes blood fats, and manufactures bile to digest dietary fats and oils. It detoxifies the blood from chemicals, drugs, and bacteria of all types. A liver clogged with poisons or excess fats cannot perform its essential duties.

The Fat Flush Program

The foods to be consumed for breakfast, lunch, and dinner are from the following food groups only. The list is restricted to whole natural foods without salt, most spices, vinegar, mustards, or herbs. (The exception is the use of small amounts of cayenne or a pinch of ginger, which may help increase metabolic rate.) These other seasonings can create water retention and yeast infections. The Two-Week Fat Flush can help diminish these problems as well, so you will find the food choices pure and simple:

Oil	*1 tablespoon twice daily*. Select organic flaxseed oil for its high Omega-3 metabolic-raising potential.
Lean protein	(up to 8 ounces per day) All varieties of fish, lean beef, veal, lamb, skinless chicken, turkey, and egg whites. Vegetarians can substitute tempeh and high-protein powders with negligible carbohydrate content.
Vegetables	Low glycemic, unlimited raw, or steamed. Choose from high-fiber selections: asparagus, green beans,

broccoli, brussels sprouts, cabbage, cauliflower, Chinese cabbage, cucumbers, eggplant, escarole, lettuce, okra, onions, parsley, green and red bell peppers, radishes, mung bean sprouts, tomatoes, watercress, zucchini, yellow squash, water chestnuts, bamboo shoots, garlic.

Fruits

2 whole portions daily. Choose from: 1 small apple, ½ grapefruit, 1 small orange, 2 medium plums, 6 large strawberries, 10 large cherries, 1 nectarine, 1 peach.

While there are many other fruits available, these choices produce the best results because they are lower on the Glycemic Index and so foster even blood sugar levels.

Long Life Cocktail

(to increase elimination) 1 teaspoon of powdered psyllium husks in 8 ounces unsweetened cranberry juice or cranberry juice sweetened with grape concentrate (available in health food stores), taken when you wake up and before bedtime. (Metamucil is a popular brand available in most pharmacies.)

Besides the Daily Diet

• With or between meals

Drink an 8-ounce cup of hot water with juice of ½ lemon twice a day to assist kidney and liver elimination.

• Breakfast and dinner

Take supplements rich in fatburning GLA. Choose from plain

GLA supplement (90 mg.) and take 2 capsules twice daily, or choose evening primrose oil (500 mg.) and take 4 capsules twice daily.

• Take a balanced multivitamin/mineral supplement.

• Take a balanced fat-burning supplement that includes some of the nutrients described in the "Fat-Burning Nutrients" chapter.

• Drink an additional 6 glasses of pure room-temperature water per day. Room temperature is best for digestion because extremely hot or extra cold or iced drinks depress gastric juices.

• Cranberry juice contains several digestive enzymes not found in other foods. To make cranberry juice yourself, here's a simple recipe: Put 1 pound of fresh cranberries into a large saucepan. Add 5 cups of water. Boil until all berries pop. Strain juice and add a touch of grape concentrate to take the edge off the tartness. Brave souls can take it straight.

• Additional water will assist in diluting the increased body wastes from the detoxification process. Spring water or filtered water is the preferred source. Distilled water is *not* recommended because it can leach minerals from the body, notably calcium, and can result in a weakened heart muscle. The water should be taken consistently throughout the day, but avoid drinking during meals so that digestive juices are not diluted. Remember that drinking adequate amounts of water is essential to weight loss.

Metabolizing stored fat into energy for the body is the liver's most important function. This water flush will allow the liver to operate at optimum potential and speed up its metabolic removal of stored fats, resulting in healthy weight loss.

Detox While Dieting

Weight loss must always accompany a detoxification program. Body fat stores environmental toxins from chemicals and pesticides in food, air, and water as well as PCBs and auto exhaust. Fat can be burned off by eating the proper foods and exercising, but the toxins are generally not burned in the usual weight-loss regimen. Unburned poisons often relocate from the shrinking fat reserves to the bloodstream, organs, and tissues, causing discomfort such as headaches and nausea. Therefore, it is imperative to deal with these toxins while dieting. My Two Week Fat Flush program does this very effectively by increasing oil, water, and exercise.

There is a twofold reason for following the daily two tablespoons of oil requirement:

1. Oil has metabolic-increasing power, and
2. Oil attracts the oil soluble poisons which have been lodged in the fatty tissues of the body and carries them out of the system for elimination.

Daily Exercise

Especially important at this time is daily moderate aerobic exercise for at least 20 to 30 minutes to keep the released toxins moving.

The Water Connection

Since water is the most natural and effective diluting agent, it is important that it be used therapeutically for cleansing. Drinking any other liquids, such as coffee, tea (even herbal teas), soft drinks, diet drinks, carbonated water, mineral water, or unsweetened fruit juices, is not recommended at this time. All of these beverages contain some type of substance that must go through a digestive process. This is exactly what you don't want.

- Drinking water before a meal takes the edge off the appetite.

- Water ensures normal bowel and kidney function to rid the body of wastes as well as stored fat.

- Drinking water alleviates fluid retention, since only when the body gets plenty of water will it release the stored water.

- Water gets rid of excess salt.

- Water helps plump the skin and prevents dehydration.

- Water helps to prevent the sagging skin conditions that often follow weight loss.

Adequate amounts of water will assist the kidneys to filter their own waste products so the liver can begin to metabolize its own waste products without having to do the kidneys' work.

Putting It All Together

A sample day from a client's diet diary on the Fat Flush Program looks like this:

Upon arising	Long Life Cocktail 30 minute brisk walk
Before Breakfast	8 ounces hot water with lemon juice
Breakfast	Egg white omelet with mushrooms and onions 2 90 mg. GLA capsules Multivitamin/mineral tablet(s) Fat burner supplement(s) 8 ounces water

Mid-morning	½ grapefruit
20 minutes before lunch	1 8-ounce glass water
Lunch	4 ounces broiled swordfish with parsley and garlic
	Large green leafy salad with chives, sprouts, shredded cabbage, and water chestnuts
	1 tablespoon flaxseed oil
	1 8-ounce glass water
Mid-afternoon	2 8-ounce glasses water
4:00 P.M.	2 plums or 1 peach
20 minutes before dinner	1 8-ounce glass water
Dinner	4 ounces baked chicken with tomatoes and onions
	4 ounces steamed asparagus
	Raw cucumber and radish-slice salad
	1 tablespoon flaxseed oil
	Fat burner supplement(s)
	2 90 mg. GLA capsules
	8 ounces hot water with lemon juice
Mid-evening	Long Life Cocktail

What It Means for You

You can use this example as a basic menu guide. Just substitute foods from the same food groups for daily variety. The time frame for the Long Life Cocktail, hot water with lemon, GLA, multivitamin/mineral supplementation, and fat burner can remain approximately the same as provided in the sample guide. You can change the fluid intake to suit your schedule if that is more convenient, of course.

A Gentle Reminder: Especially for This Two-Week Period

No herbs, spices, vinegar, mustard, or soy sauce.

No trans fats.

No alcohol.

No sugar.

No oils or fats of any kind other than the daily salad oil and the good-fat supplements.

No grains, bread, cereal, or starchy vegetables such as beans, potatoes, corn, parsnips, carrots, peas, pumpkin, or acorn or butternut squash.

No egg yolks or dairy products such as milk or cheese.

Seasonal Tune-up

This two-week cleansing diet is a marvelous body tune-up. You may want to consider doing this cleanse four times a year right before the seasons change. My patients usually will take the first two weeks of January, April, July, and October to get back on track and lose their fat.

Now you are ready for the next step.

For your convenience, there is now a Fat Flush Kit available through Uni Key at 1-800-888-4353.

The kit contains a multivitamin/mineral, a fat burner supplement, and GLA.

18

THE *BEYOND PRITIKIN* DIET PRESCRIPTION

Prepare simple meals, chew well, sup lightly.
—LEONARDO DA VINCI

Now you are ready to put all the dietary concepts of the *Beyond Pritikin* plan together in an easy-to-follow daily plan. Here is the daily Master Formula that will ensure optimum nutrition.

The *Beyond Pritikin* Diet Master Formula

1. 2 tablespoons essential-fat oil
2. 6 to 8 ounces protein
3. 4 or more vegetable servings
4. 1 to 3 fruit servings
5. 2 or more complex carbohydrate servings (starch)
6. 2 nonfat dairy servings (optional)
7. 2 90-mg. GLA supplements (4 90-mg. GLA for weight loss) twice daily
8. 1 1000-mg. Super MAXEPA twice daily
9. Balanced multivitamin/mineral supplement

Do not eat   Trans fats (margarine, vegetable shortening, refined polyunsaturated oils)

Refined carbohydrates (white flour, white sugar, cookies, candy, cake, soda)

Do not drink Alcohol

Do not compromise on trans fats, refined carbohydrates, or alcohol. These "foodless foods" can sabotage your health by blocking weight loss and prostaglandin production needed to regulate the cardiovascular, immune, and central nervous systems, as well as reproduction.

The Food Equivalents lists for essential and healthy fats, proteins, vegetables, fruits, complex carbohydrates, and dairy products (see pp. 224–231) will help you to choose the right portions for each serving of food, while reminding you of the great variety of foods available.

If you would like to follow a more specific plan, the 21-Day Master Menu is for you. The sample menus and recipes are based on the Master Formula. They are designed to omit dietary culprits such as damaged fats, excessively gluten-rich grains, fermented seasoning such as soy sauce, and the repetition of the same foods every day. By avoiding these dietary pitfalls, weight loss will be dramatic, digestion will improve, allergic edema will be eliminated, and the immune system will be strengthened.

If you are following the 21-Day Master Menu Plan, the Food Equivalents lists will also help you. You can switch any fruit or vegetable on the plan for another, provided you follow the recommended portion amounts for the substituted fruit or vegetable. For example, let's say that it is January and corn is on the menu. If you don't like frozen corn (frozen foods are allowed) but want a fresh seasonal vegetable instead, then look under the complex-carbohydrate list and find a vegetable that is in season—winter squash, for example. You can easily substitute ½ cup winter squash for the small ear of corn on the menu. Remember to choose those foods that are lower on the Index, if possible.

For practical purposes, you will find a variety of cereal choices for breakfast. Do be aware that the best choices are the whole-grain hot cereals. However, the cold cereals suggested are lower on the Glycemic Index than the puffed kind. Although there are high-fiber cold cereals now available on the market that are also lower on the Index, many of them contain aspartame and so are not recommended (such as Kellogg's All-Bran and General Mills' Fiber One).

Whichever strategy you follow (the Master Formula to create your own food plan or the suggested menus) you can achieve excellent results. You might also decide simply to use some of the recipes in your own menu plan. That's fine, too.

21-Day Master Menu Plan

Following is a 21-day menu program to get you started eating the *Beyond Pritikin* way. Each menu incorporates the nutritional information outlined in the preceding chapters. Below are just a few guidelines to be followed daily:

- Recipes noted with an asterisk (*) appear in recipe section.

- For weight loss, follow amounts given in parentheses. Others may eat as much as they want.

- Beverages with meals include 1 cup herbal tea, mineral water, or coffee substitute.

- To increase protein levels when cereal with milk is suggested for breakfast, mix 1–2 tablespoons of protein powder (which contains zero carbohydrate grams) with the milk.

- During this three week period snacks should be chosen from the 1 to 3 fruit servings (see pp. 227–228). After this time you can substitute 1 Sweet Delight serving (pp. 217–223) for one of the fruit portions.

- When the fresh fruits and vegetables mentioned are not available, frozen vegetables and fruits, or fruits canned in their own juices, are suitable substitutes.

• For those wishing to avoid milk, see p. 231 for milk substitutes.

WEEK ONE

Monday

Breakfast	2 tablespoons apple butter in (½ cup) slow-cooked oatmeal
	1 cup nonfat milk
Lunch	3 ounces canned or poached salmon with dill
	Warm asparagus
	Mixed green salad with
	*1 tablespoon Hazelnut Dressing (p. 191)
Dinner	4 ounces skinned roast turkey (white meat only)
	Baked cauliflower topped with
	*1 tablespoon Sesame Lemon Dressing (p. 193)
	(½ cup) baked winter squash with
	¼ teaspoon vanilla extract and ⅛ teaspoon cinnamon

Tuesday

Breakfast	4 halves dried apricots chopped into
	(½ cup) whole grain rye cereal and
	1 cup nonfat milk
Lunch	4 ounces lean broiled burger with sliced onions and parsley
	Green beans
	Sliced tomatoes with
	*1 tablespoon Walnut Raspberry Vinaigrette (p. 192)
Dinner	4 ounces shrimp with water chestnuts, carrots, bok choy, and bean sprouts stir-sautéed in
	*1 tablespoon Peanut Dressing with Ginger and Garlic (p. 193)
	(½ cup) Chinese rice noodles

Wednesday

Breakfast	½ banana sliced on (½ cup) cooked barley and 1 cup nonfat milk
Lunch	4 ounces curried tuna on sliced green peppers, radishes, and celery with *1 tablespoon French Olive Oil Dressing (p. 192) (½ cup) beets steamed with 2 small cinnamon sticks
Dinner	*4 ounces Chicken with Sherry Dijon (p. 203) Baked chayote squash or zucchini topped with *1 tablespoon Sesame Lemon Dressing (p. 193) *Minted Carrots and Snow Peas (p. 216)

Thursday

Breakfast	1 small nectarine or peach 2 soft- or hard-cooked eggs 1 cup nonfat milk
Lunch	*(1 cup) Sherried Black Bean Soup (p. 199) Steamed broccoli Radish and cucumber salad with *1 tablespoon Hazelnut Dressing (p. 191)
Dinner	*4 ounces Spiced Salmon Loaf (p. 208) *Bombay Curry Sauce (p. 194) Braised carrots and cabbage with ¼ teaspoon caraway seeds topped with *1 tablespoon Safflower Dressing with Papaya and Tarragon (p. 192) (½ cup) brown rice

Friday

Breakfast	*1 Baked Apple with Raisins, Cinnamon, and Nutmeg (p. 218) (1 slice) rye toast with 1 ounce tofu 1 cup nonfat milk

Lunch	3 ounces canned or broiled fresh mackerel fillets with salsa
	Sautéed red peppers and onions in white wine
	Green leafy salad with
	*1 tablespoon Sesame Lemon Dressing (p. 193)
Dinner	4 ounces broiled lamb chop with rosemary
	Grilled eggplant and tomato garnish topped with
	*1 tablespoon French Olive Oil Dressing (p. 192)
	(¾ cup) steamed green peas

Saturday

Breakfast	½ cup blueberries
	(½ cup) buckwheat groats (kasha) and
	1 cup nonfat milk
Lunch	*6 tablespoons Chickpea Sesame Pâté on (p. 196)
	(4) rye crackers with
	Sliced celery, jicama, turnips, and green peppers
Dinner	4 ounces roasted Cornish game hen
	(½ cup) wild rice and mushroom stuffing
	Steamed asparagus with lemon
	Lettuce and sliced water chestnuts with
	*1 tablespoon Safflower Dressing with Papaya and Tarragon (p. 192)

Sunday

Breakfast	1 medium sliced peach
	(½ cup) Grape-Nuts and
	1 cup nonfat milk
Lunch	*Spinach Fritatta (p. 211)
	(½ cup) cooked millet topped with
	*1 tablespoon Perfect Pesto (p. 194)
Dinner	*Five Spice Chicken and Vegetable Sauté (p. 207)
	Leafy green salad with
	*1 tablespoon Hazelnut Dressing (p. 191)

WEEK TWO

Monday

Breakfast	½ cup pineapple chunks with ½ cup nonfat cottage cheese 1 cup nonfat milk
Lunch	*(1 cup) Greek Lentil Soup (p. 199) Endive and bermuda onion salad with *1 tablespoon French Olive Oil Dressing (p. 192) (1 slice) whole-wheat toast
Dinner	*4 ounces Baked Salmon in Wine with Savory (p. 208) *Fresh Tomato Piquant (p. 194) Green beans almondine *Coleslaw with Anise, Caraway, and Poppy Seeds mixed with (p. 216) *1 tablespoon Safflower Dressing with Papaya and Tarragon (p. 192)

Tuesday

Breakfast	2 tablespoons unsweetened raspberry preserves with 1 cup nonfat yogurt
Lunch	2 hard-cooked eggs on raw spinach with Celery, artichoke hearts, and roasted red peppers *1 tablespoon Walnut Raspberry Vinaigrette (p. 192)
Dinner	4 ounces broiled lamb patty with ⅛ teaspoon dried mint (¼ cup) sweet potato Swiss chard sautéed in *1 tablespoon French Olive Oil Dressing (p. 192)

Wednesday

Breakfast	1 dried fig chopped in (½ cup) slow-cooked oatmeal and 1 cup nonfat milk

Lunch	*(1 cup) Vegetable Bean Soup with Oregano and Basil (p. 201)
	½ cup fresh goat cheese on radicchio
	*1 tablespoon Sesame Lemon Dressing (p. 193)
Dinner	4 ounces veal strips
	*Ratatouille (p. 215)
	(½ cup) acorn squash

Thursday

Breakfast	½ cup blueberries in
	(2) buckwheat pancakes
	1 cup nonfat milk
Lunch	*Gazpacho or vegetable soup (p. 200)
	(½ cup) grated raw beets and daikon with
	2 ounces cubed tofu with
	*1 tablespoon Hazelnut Dressing (p. 191)
Dinner	*Eskimo Salad Niçoise (p. 207)
	Steamed broccoli

Friday

Breakfast	1 small chopped apple in
	(½ cup) cooked oat bran
	1 cup nonfat milk
Lunch	*(1 cup) Split Pea and Yam Soup (p. 201)
	Spinach salad with 2 sliced hard-cooked eggs
	*1 tablespoon Safflower Dressing with Papaya and Tarragon (p. 192)
Dinner	*4 ounces Cajun Cod (p. 202)
	Okra and zucchini sautéed in
	*1 tablespoon French Olive Oil Dressing (p. 192)
	Cucumber spears

Saturday

Breakfast	½ cup unsweetened cranberry juice
	(1 slice) whole-grain toast with
	1 tablespoon sesame butter
	1 cup nonfat milk

Lunch   *6 tablespoons Jack's Party Pâté on (p. 197)
               (2) rice cakes with
               Celery, jicama, and carrot sticks

Dinner   4 ounces flank steak with
               *Horseradish Sauce with Dill (p. 196)
               Steamed peas, onions, and green beans
               Bean sprouts, bamboo shoots, and red peppers
                  stir-sautéed in
               *1 tablespoon Peanut Dressing with Ginger and
                  Garlic (p. 193)

Sunday

Breakfast   ½ cup blueberries with
               (½ cup) Wheatena
               1 cup nonfat milk

Lunch   *(1 cup) Sherried Black Bean Soup (p. 199)
               ½ cup feta cheese crumbled in
               Green leafy salad with
               *1 tablespoon French Olive Oil Dressing (p. 192)

Dinner   *4 ounces Halibut Shrimp Kabob Marinated in
                  Galliano, Garlic, and Chili (p. 210)
               Red and green cabbage with
               ¼ teaspoon poppyseed stir-sautéed in
               *1 tablespoon Peanut Dressing with Ginger and
                  Garlic (p. 193)

WEEK THREE

Monday

Breakfast   2 tablespoons unsweetened blackberry fruit
                  preserves on
               ½ cup nonfat cottage cheese
               *(2) Magic Muffins (p. 219)

Lunch   *6 tablespoons Sweetheart Pâté with (p. 198)
               Sliced raw mushrooms, cauliflower, and broc-
                  coli
               Steamed artichoke dipped in
               *1 tablespoon Sesame Lemon Dressing (p. 193)

Dinner	4 ounces veal strips cooked in white wine
	Brussels sprouts
	(3½ ounces sliced) Jerusalem artichoke (sun-chokes) topped with
	*1 tablespoon Safflower Dressing with Papaya and Tarragon (p. 192)

Tuesday

Breakfast	2 tablespoons raisins with
	(½ cup) cooked barley or barley flakes
	1 cup nonfat milk
Lunch	Vegetable broth
	3 ounces shredded crab in small avocado with juice of ½ lemon
	Sweet onion and celery salad
Dinner	4 ounces broiled chicken with lime juice
	(1 small) corn on the cob
	Leeks and zucchini stir-sautéed in
	*1 tablespoon French Olive Oil Dressing (p. 192)

Wednesday

Breakfast	2 medium dried prunes chopped in
	(½ cup) whole rye cereal
	1 cup nonfat milk
Lunch	*4 ounces Grilled Tuna (p. 209)
	*Chili Mayonnaise (p. 195)
	Warm asparagus
	Spinach and pimento salad with rice vinegar
Dinner	*Old-Fashioned Brisket of Beef with Vegetables and Gravy (p. 206)
	Sliced tomatoes with
	*1 tablespoon Hazelnut Dressing (p. 191)

Thursday

Breakfast	½ banana
	(½ cup) buckwheat groats (kasha) and
	1 cup nonfat milk

Lunch	4 ounces sardines with

Lunch   4 ounces sardines with
            Chopped tomato, parsley, and scallions in
            *1 tablespoon Walnut Raspberry Vinaigrette
                (p. 192)
            Baked cauliflower with lemon juice
Dinner   *4 ounces Mediterranean Meatballs with
                (p. 203)
            Spaghetti squash
            Green beans with
            ½ teaspoon toasted sesame seeds
            (1 small) corn on the cob with
            *1 tablespoon Sesame Lemon Dressing (p. 193)

Friday

Breakfast   2 tablespoons apple butter with
            (½ cup) slow-cooked oatmeal and
            1 cup nonfat milk
Lunch   *3 Salmon Croquettes with (p. 204)
            *Herbed Hollandaise (p. 195)
            Grated daikon, carrot, and onion salad
            *1 tablespoon Safflower Dressing with Papaya
                and Tarragon (p. 192)
Dinner   *1 Stuffed Peppers Oreganato (p. 205)
            Swiss chard sautéed in
            *1 tablespoon Peanut Dressing with Ginger and
                Garlic (p. 193)
            (½ cup) succotash

Saturday

Breakfast   1 small sliced peach with
            (½ cup) Grape-Nuts and
            1 cup nonfat milk
Lunch   4 ounces tuna with
            Juice of ½ lemon
            (2) rice cakes
            *Coleslaw with Anise, Caraway, and Poppy
                Seeds (p. 216)
            *1 tablespoon Safflower Dressing with Papaya
                and Tarragon (p. 192)

Dinner   4 ounces shrimp sautéed in white wine and
                    parsley
                Steamed yellow squash
                *Ratatouille (p. 215)

Sunday

Breakfast   ¾ cup strawberries
                *Laced Artichoke Omelet (p. 210)
                (1 slice) rye toast
                1 cup nonfat milk

Lunch   4 ounces lean broiled turkey burger with
                    ⅛ teaspoon fennel
                Steamed green beans
                Chopped parsley, onion, and tomato salad
                *1 tablespoon French Olive Oil Dressing (p. 192)

Dinner   *4 ounces Lemon-Baked Halibut with (p. 205)
                *Garlic Roasted Peppers and Anchovies (p. 215)
                (¼ cup) yams
                Grated jicama on romaine lettuce with cham-
                    pagne vinegar

Recipes

SALAD DRESSINGS AND SAUCES

Hazelnut Dressing

Nut oils are so highly flavored that they make truly mem-
orable salad dressings. A little bit of oil goes a long way
in flavor.

Serves 8 (1 tablespoon = 1 serving)

  ½ cup hazelnut oil
  2 tablespoons balsamic vinegar or cider vinegar
  ½ teaspoon salt (optional)
  ⅛–¼ teaspoon freshly ground black pepper

Place all ingredients in a small covered jar. Shake well.
Refrigerate.

Safflower Dressing with Papaya and Tarragon

Safflower oil is the lightest and most mildly flavored oil
of all. It is also the most commonly used in diets because
it is the highest in cis-linoleic acid, which can convert
into fat-burning GLA. This dressing goes well with salads
and fish.

Serves 8 (1 tablespoon = 1 serving)

½ cup safflower oil
1 tablespoon papaya juice concentrate
1 tablespoon finely chopped sweet onion
½ teaspoon tarragon
¼ teaspoon salt (optional)

Place all ingredients in a small covered jar. Shake well.
Refrigerate.

Walnut Raspberry Vinaigrette

Another nut oil winner, walnut oil lends itself nicely to
exotic vinegar accompaniments.

Serves 8 (1 tablespoon = 1 serving)

½ cup walnut oil
2 tablespoons raspberry vinegar
½ teaspoon salt (optional)
⅛–¼ teaspoon freshly ground black pepper

Place all ingredients in a small covered jar. Shake well.
Refrigerate.

French Olive Oil Dressing

Whether used as a salad dressing or to sauté, this basic
French-style dressing is a favorite.

Serves 8 (1 tablespoon = 1 serving)

½ cup extra virgin olive oil
2 tablespoons fresh lemon juice
1 teaspoon Dijon mustard
¼ teaspoon salt (optional)

Put all ingredients in a small covered jar. Shake vigorously for 30 seconds and refrigerate. Remove from the refrigerator at least 1 hour before serving to liquefy the oil.

Peanut Dressing with Ginger and Garlic

Like French Olive Oil Dressing, this can also be used for sautéing as well as on salads.

Serves 8 (1 tablespoon = 1 serving)

½ cup peanut oil
1½ tablespoons finely chopped fresh ginger
1 tablespoon chopped parsley
1 garlic clove, minced
¼ teaspoon salt (optional)

Put all ingredients in a small covered jar. Shake well and refrigerate. Remove at least 1 hour before serving to liquefy the oil.

Sesame Lemon Dressing

Sesame oil has a delicate yet distinctive taste that imparts a nutty flavor to all its companion vegetables.

Serves 8 (1 tablespoon = 1 serving)

½ cup light sesame oil
1 tablespoon fresh lemon juice
½ teaspoon grated fresh lemon zest
¼ teaspoon salt (optional)
½ teaspoon dried dill

Combine all ingredients in a small covered jar. Shake well. Refrigerate.

Perfect Pesto

A delicious dressing or sauce high in the beneficial Omega-3s. My clients prefer Barlean's or Spectrum flaxseed oil.

Serves 8 (1 tablespoon = 1 serving)

    2 cups packed fresh basil
    ½ cup freshly grated parmesan cheese
    ¼ cup olive oil
    ¼ cup organic flaxseed oil
    2 cloves garlic, minced
    1 handful pine nuts

In blender or food processor blend all ingredients until smoothly pureed. Add a touch of olive oil to thin to taste.

Bombay Curry Sauce

This sauce enhances all fish dishes.

Serves 4 (3 tablespoons = 1 serving)

    1 onion, chopped
    1 green cooking apple (such as Granny Smith),
        chopped but not peeled
    1 tablespoon butter
    2 teaspoons curry powder
    1 tablespoon arrowroot
    ½ cup nonfat milk
    ½ teaspoon salt (optional)

Sauté onion and apple in butter until tender. Add curry powder and simmer 2 minutes, stirring frequently. Add arrowroot. Mix thoroughly. Add milk and salt (optional), stirring constantly until mixture starts to bubble. Remove from heat.

Fresh Tomato Piquant

This topping adds a refreshing accent to fish and baked potatoes.

Serves 4 (1 heaping tablespoon = 1 serving, but can be eaten in unlimited amounts)

 4 tablespoons chopped cilantro
 ½ green pepper, chopped
 1 ripe tomato, seeded and chopped
 3 tablespoons finely chopped sweet onion
 ½ teaspoon salt (optional)

Combine all ingredients and toss lightly.

Chili Mayonnaise

A homemade real mayonnaise that is perfect with fish.

Makes about 1¼ cups (1 tablespoon = 1 serving)

 3 egg yolks
 ¼ teaspoon salt (optional)
 3 tablespoons fresh lemon juice
 1 cup virgin olive oil
 1 teaspoon chili powder

Combine the egg yolks, salt, and lemon juice, whisking constantly. Add in the oil slowly until the consistency is smooth. Stir in chili powder. Store in the refrigerator.

Herbed Hollandaise

This light version of the traditional hollandaise is tasty and more nutritious than the original. It is delicious with mild-flavored fish such as sole and salmon, and highlights all vegetables.

Serves 4 (4 tablespoons = 1 serving)

 1½ teaspoons arrowroot
 ¾ cup water
 3 tablespoons fresh lemon juice
 ½ teaspoon salt (optional)
 ⅛ teaspoon cayenne pepper
 1 whole egg, beaten

1 egg yolk, beaten
2 tablespoons mixed chopped fresh herbs
   (parsley, thyme, chervil, tarragon, and basil)

Dissolve arrowroot in water in saucepan. Bring to a boil
and cook 1 minute. Reduce heat. Add lemon juice, salt
(optional), and cayenne. Combine whole egg with the
yolk. Pour mixture into beaten eggs, whisking constantly
with a wire whisk. Return to saucepan and cook over
low heat, stirring constantly. Remove the sauce from the
heat and fold in fresh herbs.

Horseradish Sauce with Dill

An interesting alternative to prepared horseradish, this
sauce can be spooned over lean beef or used as a dip for
crispy fresh vegetables.

Serves 4 (4 tablespoons = 1 serving)

   ½ cup nonfat yogurt
   ½ cup nonfat cottage cheese
   ½ teaspoon powdered horseradish or
      2 teaspoons prepared horseradish
   ½ teaspoon Worcestershire sauce
   ½ teaspoon snipped fresh dill
   ¼ teaspoon salt (optional)

Place all ingredients in a blender or food processor.
Blend until smooth. Make sure the cottage cheese is
liquefied into a sauce consistency.

PÂTÉS

Chickpea Sesame Pâté

Enjoy this pâté with crackers for a quick meal or serve
as a Mediterranean hors d'oeuvre for entertaining. Versatile Chickpea Sesame Pâté also makes a delicious sandwich filler.

Serves 4 (6 tablespoons = 1 serving)

1½ cups cooked or canned garbanzos
  (chickpeas), drained, reserving liquid
3 tablespoons chopped onion
3 tablespoons chopped parsley
1 large garlic clove, minced
1 teaspoon dried basil
½ teaspoon dried oregano
¼ teaspoon ground cumin
1 tablespoon sesame seed butter
¼ cup sesame seeds
¼ teaspoon salt (optional)
2 tablespoons fresh lemon juice
1 tablespoon liquid from chickpeas

Place all ingredients in food processor or blender. Blend well. Add more liquid if needed when using a blender. Pâté should be thick enough to spread.

Jack's Party Pâté

This is a unique dip, with mysterious ingredients that will leave everyone guessing. (Omit anchovies if on a sodium-restricted diet.)

Serves 8 (6 tablespoons = 1 serving)

2 13-ounce cans water-packed tuna, rinsed,
  drained, reserving liquid for blender
1 8-ounce can oysters, rinsed and drained
1 2-ounce can anchovy fillets, well rinsed and
  drained
1 garlic clove, minced
2 tablespoons chopped parsley
¼ teaspoon dried dill
½ teaspoon Dijon mustard
¼ teaspoon dried horseradish or 1 teaspoon
  prepared horseradish
1 teaspoon fresh lemon juice

1 teaspoon Bakon Yeast (a brand name yeast
available in health food stores)

Place all ingredients in food processor or blender and
blend until smooth. Add more liquid if needed when
using a blender.

Sweetheart Pâté

With crackers or raw vegetables, this pâté is also good
for company.

Serves 4 (6 tablespoons = 1 serving)

1 15½-ounce can salmon, bones and skin
    removed, rinsed but not drained, reserving
    liquid
2 tablespoons fresh lemon juice
1 teaspoon dried dill or 1 tablespoon fresh dill
1 tablespoon agar-agar (seaweed gelatin)*
2 tablespoons salmon liquid
½ cup chopped sweet onion
¼ cup chopped fresh parsley
1 tablespoon capers, rinsed and drained

Place salmon, lemon juice and dill in food processor or
blender. Blend for 10 seconds. Dissolve agar-agar in
salmon liquid in a saucepan and bring to a boil. Add
dissolved agar-agar to salmon mixture. Stir in onion,
parsley, and capers.

SOUPS

In any climate, and any season, soups are satisfying liquid meals. Whether hot or cold they provide good nutrition and round out any dietary plan. Basic stocks from
chicken, fish, and vegetables can be used to enhance nutritional value when cooking main dishes, vegetables,
and/or grains.

*Agar-agar is available at health food stores.

Sherried Black Bean Soup

An exotic variation of a traditional staple.

Serves 4 (1 cup = 1 serving)

    1 cup dried black beans, washed and soaked in
        4 cups water overnight, then drained
    4 cups water
    1 tablespoon olive oil
    2 tablespoons fresh lemon juice
    1 onion, chopped
    1 carrot, chopped
    1 celery stalk with leaves, chopped
    1 garlic clove, minced
    2 tablespoons chopped fresh parsley
    1/8 teaspoon cayenne
    3/4 teaspoon salt (optional)
    4 tablespoons sherry
    1 thinly sliced lemon for garnish
    1 hard-cooked chopped egg for garnish

Place drained beans in covered pot. Add 4 cups water. Bring to boil and simmer. Add olive oil and lemon juice. Cook 2 to 3 hours until beans are tender. Add onion, carrot, celery, garlic, parsley, cayenne, salt (optional), and sherry. Simmer an additional 30 to 45 minutes until vegetables are tender. Garnish each bowl of soup with lemon slice and chopped egg.

Greek Lentil Soup

The unusual spices give this soup a Mediterranean taste.

Serves 4 (1 cup = 1 serving)

    1 cup lentils, washed and soaked in 4 cups water
        overnight
    3 cups water
    1 tablespoon olive oil
    1 tablespoon fresh lemon juice

1 onion, chopped
1 carrot, chopped
½ cup chopped green pepper
1 celery stalk with leaves, chopped
1 garlic clove, minced
2 tablespoons chopped fresh parsley
½ bay leaf
¾ teaspoon salt (optional)
½ teaspoon mustard seed
½ teaspoon ground cumin
2 tablespoons finely chopped green onions for
    garnish

Place drained lentils in 3 cups water in covered pot. Bring to boil and simmer. Add olive oil and lemon juice. Cook 30 minutes until lentils are tender. Add onion, carrot, green pepper, celery, garlic, parsley, bay leaf, salt (optional), mustard seed, and cumin. Simmer covered an additional 20 to 30 minutes until vegetables are tender.

Gazpacho

A Spanish cold-soup favorite from south of the border for hot weather. Use garden-fresh ingredients for best flavor.

Serves 4 (1 cup = 1 serving)

4 tomatoes, peeled, seeded, and coarsely
    chopped
½ cup chopped sweet onion
½ cucumber, peeled, seeded, and chopped
½ green pepper, seeded and chopped
1 garlic clove, minced
2 tablespoons olive oil
3 tablespoons red wine vinegar
½ cup ice water
½ teaspoon salt (optional)

2 tablespoons chopped fresh basil or fresh
parsley

Place all ingredients in a food processor or blender. Blend until smooth. Serve in chilled bowls.

Split Pea and Yam Soup

The addition of a yam or sweet potato gives a distinctively sweet flavor to this tasty split pea soup.

Serves 4 (1 cup = 1 serving)

1 cup split peas, washed and soaked in 4 cups
water overnight
3 cups water
1 tablespoon olive oil
1 onion, chopped
1 carrot, chopped
1 celery stalk with leaves, chopped
1 small yam or sweet potato, peeled and cubed
1 garlic clove, minced
2 tablespoons chopped fresh parsley
½ bay leaf
¾ teaspoon salt (optional)
¼ teaspoon caraway seeds

Place drained split peas and 3 cups water in covered pot. Bring to boil and simmer. Add olive oil. Cook 30 minutes until split peas are soft. Add onion, carrot, celery, yam (or sweet potato), garlic, parsley, bay leaf, salt (optional) and caraway seeds. Simmer an additional 20 to 30 minutes until vegetables are tender.

Vegetable Bean Soup with Oregano and Basil

A good basic soup!

Serves 4 (1 cup = 1 serving)

1 cup dried white beans, washed, sorted, and
soaked in 4 cups water overnight

4 cups water
1 tablespoon olive oil
1 tablespoon fresh lemon juice
1 onion, chopped
1 carrot, chopped
1 celery stalk with leaves, chopped
1 garlic clove, chopped
1 tablespoon chopped fresh parsley
½ bay leaf
¾ teaspoon salt (optional)
½ teaspoon dried oregano
¼ teaspoon dried basil

Place drained beans in covered pot. Add 4 cups water. Bring to boil and simmer. Add olive oil and lemon juice. Cook 2 to 3 hours until beans are tender. Add onion, carrot, celery, garlic, parsley, bay leaf, salt (optional), oregano, and basil. Simmer an additional 30 to 45 minutes until vegetables are tender.

MAIN EVENTS

The oil portion in these recipes is controlled for those who are following the 21-Day Master Menu Plan. If you're not using the Master Menus, additional oil can be used—1 tablespoon per person per meal—to add flavor and tenderness to any of the Main Events. Add the oil after cooking unless it is olive, canola, or peanut oil, which can be used in cooking or for sautéing.

Cajun Cod

A spicy twist for a mild-mannered fish!

Serves 4 (4 ounces cooked fish = 1 serving)

1 medium onion, chopped
1 green pepper, chopped
1 garlic clove, minced
1 teaspoon butter

2 fresh tomatoes, seeded and chopped
½ cup red wine
¼ teaspoon thyme
½ teaspoon cayenne pepper
4 5-ounce cod fillets
2 tablespoons fresh lemon juice

Sauté onion, green pepper, and garlic in butter until tender. Add tomatoes, wine, thyme, and cayenne. Bring to a boil. Add cod, reduce heat, cover, and simmer about 10 minutes or until fish flakes. Add lemon juice just before serving.

Chicken with Sherry Dijon

Easy and elegant, this tasty main dish can be served with minimum effort.

Serves 4 (4 ounces cooked chicken = 1 serving)

2 whole chicken breasts (2 pounds chicken),
    skinned and halved
½ cup Dijon mustard
4 tablespoons sherry

Preheat oven to 350°. Rub chicken breasts with ¼ cup mustard. Place chicken in covered baking pan. Add sherry to remaining ¼ cup mustard for basting. Bake chicken 45 minutes, basting frequently with the Sherry Dijon.

Mediterranean Meatballs

The combination of meatballs with spaghetti squash provides an interesting alternative to the traditional pasta dish, without the pasta!

Serves 4 (4 meatballs = 1 serving)

1 pound lean ground round
⅓ cup oat bran
1 egg, beaten

    ½ teaspoon salt (optional)
    1 tablespoon chopped fresh parsley
    ½ teaspoon ground cumin
    ⅛ teaspoon ground allspice
    ⅛ teaspoon cayenne
    1 15-ounce can chicken broth (Health Valley
       preferred)
    4 tablespoons instant potatoes (Barbara's
       preferred)

Preheat broiler. In mixing bowl, combine ground meat, oat bran, egg, salt (optional), parsley, cumin, allspice, and cayenne. Form into 16 balls. Broil 14 inches from heat for 8 minutes. Turn and broil another 4 minutes.

Heat chicken broth and thicken with instant potatoes to make a sauce. Season to taste. Add meatballs to sauce and serve over spaghetti squash.

Salmon Croquettes

A quick way to get your Omega-3s. Herbed Hollandaise is the sauce of choice.

Serves 4 (3 croquettes = 1 serving)

    1 15½-ounce can salmon, drained, bones and
       skin removed, and flaked
    ¼ cup crushed cornflakes (salt- and sugar-free)
    ⅓ cup finely chopped onion
    ⅓ cup finely chopped fresh parsley
    2 tablespoons fresh lemon juice
    1 egg, beaten
    ⅓ cup crushed cornflakes
    4 lemon wedges for garnish

Preheat oven to 350°. Combine salmon with ¼ cup crushed cornflakes, onion, parsley, lemon juice, and beaten egg. Shape into 12 croquettes. Roll in the ⅓ cup crushed cornflakes. Bake for 20 to 30 minutes. Serve with lemon wedge garnish.

Stuffed Peppers Oreganato

A healthy touch of bran for an old favorite. You can literally feel your oats!

Serves 4 (1 stuffed pepper = 1 serving)

> 1 pound ground round beef
> ½ onion, finely chopped
> ⅓ cup oat bran
> ½ teaspoon salt (optional)
> ½ teaspoon dried oregano
> ¼ teaspoon paprika
> 5 drops Tabasco
> ⅛ teaspoon cayenne
> 2 large green bell peppers, halved, seeds and
>   membranes removed
> ½ cup chicken broth

Preheat oven to 350°. Mix ground round, onion, and oat bran. Add salt (optional), oregano, paprika, Tabasco, and cayenne. Fill pepper halves with this mixture. Place stuffed peppers in baking dish with chicken broth and cover. Bake for 45 minutes to 1 hour. Serve with broth spooned over peppers.

Lemon-Baked Halibut

An easy-to-prepare dish in which the delicate fish flavor prevails.

Serves 4 (4 ounces cooked fish = 1 serving)

> 4 5-ounce halibut fillets
> 1 tablespoon finely minced garlic
> 1 tablespoon grated fresh lemon zest
> ⅛ teaspoon salt (optional)

Preheat oven to 350°. Place fillets in baking dish. Sprinkle with garlic and lemon zest. Lightly salt (optional). Cover and bake for 15 to 20 minutes, or until fish is completely white and flakes.

Old-Fashioned Brisket of Beef Dinner
with Vegetables and Gravy

This recipe is an East Coast favorite, perfect for a cold winter's day.

Serves 4.

> 1 3-pound beef brisket, all visible fat removed
> 2 cups water
> 1 large onion, stuck with 3 whole cloves
> 1 large carrot, cut in chunks
> 2 celery stalks with leaves, cut in 1-inch pieces
> 1 bay leaf
> 3 garlic cloves, peeled and pressed
> 1 teaspoon salt (optional)
> 1 teaspoon freshly ground pepper
> 4 small red potatoes
> 4 carrots, cut in chunks
> 4 small whole onions, peeled
> 4 small turnips, peeled (if available)
> 1 small head cabbage, quartered
> 1 teaspoon powdered horseradish or
>   4 teaspoons prepared horseradish

In a large kettle, sear beef brisket over medium heat until browned. Pour off fat. Add water, cloved onion, the biggest carrot, celery, bay leaf, garlic, salt (optional), and pepper. Cover, bring to a boil, and simmer 2½ hours. Remove vegetables and bay leaf and reserve for gravy.

Add potatoes and remaining vegetables in order given. Sprinkle cabbage with powdered horseradish (or spread with prepared horseradish). Cover and simmer an additional 1½ to 2 hours until meat is tender and vegetables are cooked but not soggy.

To prepare gravy: Add vegetables and bay leaf set aside earlier and mash them into meat broth. Bring to boil and reduce to desired consistency. Adjust seasonings to taste and remove bay leaf. To serve, slice cooked brisket across the grain in 1-inch slices. Place on large platter and surround with vegetables. Spoon gravy over brisket.

Eskimo Salad Niçoise

This salad is an Omega-3 adaptation of the classic French salad.

Serves 4

> 4 small red potatoes, unpeeled, steamed, cooled, and sliced
> 2 cups fresh green beans, steamed, cooled, and sliced
> 1 small sweet onion, thinly sliced into rings
> 24 French or Niçoise olives, pitted
> 2 tablespoons chopped fresh parsley
> 4 4-ounce cans water-packed sardines, rinsed and drained
> 3 tablespoons fresh lemon juice
> 4 tablespoons of French Olive Oil Dressing (p. 192)
> Red leaf or butter lettuce leaves for serving
> 2 hard-cooked eggs, shelled and quartered into wedges for garnish

Combine potatoes, green beans, onion rings, olives, and parsley in a large salad bowl. Add sardines, sprinkled with lemon juice. Toss lightly with dressing. Arrange salad on lettuce leaves. Place egg wedges around the salad. Serve chilled.

Five Spice Chicken and Vegetable Sauté

Crisp and brightly colored, this stir-sauté combination is an enjoyable Main Event.

Serves 4 (4 ounces cooked chicken = 1 serving)

> ½ cup chicken broth
> 2 whole chicken breasts (2 pounds chicken), skinned, boned, and cut into ½-inch pieces

2 stalks broccoli, lightly steamed and diagonally
   sliced
½ red pepper, sliced
2 carrots, lightly steamed and diagonally sliced
2 yellow crookneck squash, diagonally sliced
   (optional)
¼ cup sliced onion
¼ cup canned water chestnuts, drained and
   sliced
1 tablespoon chopped fresh parsley
¼ teaspoon Chinese five spice powder
2 cups cooked brown rice

Heat chicken broth in a skillet or wok. Add chicken and
cook until tender. Remove chicken from broth and set
aside. Add broccoli, red pepper, carrots, squash, onion,
and water chestnuts. Stir and cook 2 to 3 minutes. Add
parsley, Chinese five spice powder, and rice. Return
cooked chicken to mixture. Stir until thoroughly heated.

Baked Salmon in Wine with Savory

This salmon is particularly good with the Fresh Tomato
Piquant (p. 194).

Serves 4 (4 ounces cooked fish = 1 serving)

4 5-ounce salmon fillets
½ cup white wine or vermouth
½ teaspoon dried savory leaves
4 sprigs cilantro or parsley for garnish

Preheat oven to 350°. Place salmon in baking dish with
wine. Sprinkle savory on fish. Cover and bake about 20
minutes, or until fish is completely pink and flakes.
Spoon remaining liquid over salmon for more flavor.
Garnish with cilantro or parsley.

Spiced Salmon Loaf

Tuna can easily be substituted for salmon in this recipe.
You can be creative with your seasonings by adding, for

example, a dash of dry mustard, curry powder, or celery seeds in addition to the seasonings already given in the recipe. Dress up your loaf with Bombay Curry Sauce (p. 194).

Serves 4 (4 ounces = 1 serving)

> 1 15½-ounce can salmon, drained, bones and
>   skin removed, and flaked
> ½ cup chopped onion
> ½ cup chopped celery
> 2 tablespoons fresh lemon juice
> 1 teaspoon dried dill
> 1½ teaspoons Worcestershire sauce
> 4 drops Tabasco
> ¼ cup oat bran
> 2 eggs, beaten
> 1 teaspoon butter

Preheat oven to 350°. Combine flaked salmon with onion, celery, lemon juice, and dill in mixing bowl. Add remaining seasonings. Stir in the oat bran. Blend in eggs. Pour into buttered loaf pan and bake for 45 minutes.

Grilled Tuna

Because of tuna's distinct flavor and meaty bite, it is best prepared simply with a zesty sauce. Chili Mayonnaise (p. 195) is a piquant choice.

Serves 4 (4 ounces cooked fish = 1 serving)

> 4 5-ounce fresh tuna steaks
> 4 tablespoons white wine

Preheat broiler. Place tuna on baking pan and spoon on wine. Broil about 6 inches from heat until fish is opaque, about 6 minutes. Turn fish over and broil until fish is firm and flakes.

Halibut Shrimp Kabob Marinated in
Galliano, Garlic, and Chili

Company fare. Marinate these kabobs overnight in the refrigerator for fullest flavor.

Serves 4 (4 ounces cooked seafood = 1 serving)

1 pound halibut, cut in 1-inch cubes
8 medium shrimp, peeled and rinsed
2 medium zucchini, cut in ½-inch slices
1 onion, cut in 1-inch cubes
2 tablespoons Galliano wine
1 clove garlic, minced
Juice of 1 lemon
1 tablespoon grated fresh lemon zest
⅛ teaspoon salt (optional)
½ teaspoon chili powder

4 large (or 8 small) bamboo skewers

Thread halibut and shrimp onto skewers, alternating with zucchini and onion cubes. In a bowl, mix Galliano wine, garlic, lemon juice, lemon zest, salt, and chili powder. Marinate for at least 1 hour in refrigerator. Brush skewers with marinade and broil 4 inches away from the heat until cooked on all sides, about 15 minutes.

Laced Artichoke Omelet

Another breakfast or brunch favorite. The wine gives a heady flavor that spikes any appetite.

Serves 4

2 large cooked artichokes, leaves scraped,
    bottoms coarsely chopped
1 teaspoon butter
8 eggs, beaten
4 tablespoons water

8 teaspoons white wine
½ teaspoon oregano
¼ teaspoon salt (optional)
⅛ teaspoon pepper

Sauté artichoke pieces in butter until lightly browned. Mix eggs with water, wine, oregano, salt, and pepper. Add to artichokes and cook over medium heat until eggs are set.

Spinach Fritatta

Ideal for breakfast or brunch.

Serves 4

6 eggs, beaten
½ cup nonfat cottage cheese
1½ cups fresh or frozen spinach, chopped and
    firmly packed
2 scallions, thinly sliced
1 teaspoon dried basil or 2 tablespoons fresh
    basil
¼ teaspoon salt (optional)
⅛ teaspoon grated nutmeg
1 teaspoon butter

Preheat oven to 350°. Combine eggs, cottage cheese, spinach, scallions, and seasonings. Melt butter in large skillet. Add egg mixture and cook over medium heat for 3 minutes. Place in oven and bake an additional 10 minutes or until set.

Vegetables

When freshly crisped for salad or lightly sautéed as a side dish, vegetables are full of natural flavor and texture. They are good fiber sources that can lower cholesterol and protect against colon cancer. Leafy greens and deep yellow vegetables are rich in vitamins A and C and also provide important minerals such as magnesium, potassium, and iron. From tangy Swiss chard to velvety sweet butternut squash, vegetables are taking on a new style. Edible blossoms such as nasturtiums and petite rose petals—unsprayed, of course—are turning up on gourmet salad plates. You can make any vegetable a specialty item by adorning it with a special dressing, sprinkling on fresh herbs, or adding your favorite sauce.

We are surrounded with increasingly exotic vegetables in even the most ordinary supermarkets. The wider variety now available means that your menus are limited only by your creativity. You can add brand-new accents to even your most basic dishes. Some of the new favorites are radicchio (Italian red chicory), sugar snap peas, radish sprouts, bok choy (Chinese mustard cabbage), shiitake mushrooms, baby eggplants, fennel, Vidalia and Walla Walla onions (white and sugar sweet), and chayote squash (known as the starchless biblical squash). In salads or soups, steamed, braised, or stir-sautéed, you can enjoy these vegetables in almost infinite ways. As a colorful puree, any vegetable can perk up your menu quite effortlessly and tastefully.

All vegetables are part of the Master Menu Plan. The amounts of the more starchy ones (such as corn, peas, and potatoes) should initially be limited until the fat burner is working at optimum metabolic strength (usually three weeks on the healthful oils). After the three-week period, both starchy vegetables and grains (such as rice and millet) can be increased.

Timetable for Steaming Fresh Vegetables

Vegetables should be steamed in a stainless steel steamer or colander over boiling water in a covered pot. Taste is enhanced when vegetables are still firm and crunchy after the steaming. The following timetable was designed with this in mind.

Vegetable	Steaming Time
Artichokes	
Globe, whole	45 minutes
Jerusalem or sunchokes, whole	7–10 minutes
Asparagus	
Whole	7–12 minutes
Tips	6–10 minutes
Beans	
Lima	20–30 minutes
Green	8–12 minutes
Wax or yellow	8–12 minutes
Beet greens	3–5 minutes
Beets	
Whole	20–25 minutes
¼-inch slices	3–5 minutes
Broccoli	
Stalks, split	8–10 minutes
Brussels sprouts	8–12 minutes
Cabbage	
Green, quartered	5–7 minutes
Green, shredded	3 minutes
Red, shredded	3 minutes
Carrots	
Whole	15–20 minutes
¼-inch slices	8–12 minutes
Cauliflower	
Whole	20–25 minutes
Florets	7–10 minutes
Celery	
Whole	8–12 minutes
Diced	3–7 minutes

Chard, Swiss	3–5 minutes
Corn	
On cob	5–8 minutes
Kernels	3–5 minutes
Eggplant	
Sliced	8–10 minutes
Kale	3–7 minutes
Kohlrabi	
Whole	10–15 minutes
Sliced	3–7 minutes
Okra	
Whole	10–12 minutes
Sliced	3–6 minutes
Onions, pearl	5–8 minutes
Parsnips	
Whole	13–17 minutes
¼-inch slices	7–10 minutes
Peas, green	3–8 minutes
Potatoes, sweet	
Whole	20–30 minutes
½-inch slices	7–10 minutes
Potatoes, White	
Whole	20–30 minutes
½-inch slices	7–10 minutes
Snow peas (pea pods)	3–5 minutes
Spinach	3–5 minutes
Squash, summer	
Whole	15–25 minutes
¼-inch slices	8–10 minutes
Squash, winter	
Whole	20–30 minutes
¼-inch slices	7–10 minutes
Tomatoes	
Whole	5–8 minutes
½-inch slices	3–5 minutes

Turnips

Whole	12–18 minutes
½-inch slices	3–6 minutes

Zucchini

Whole	8–12 minutes
¼-inch slices	3–6 minutes

Ratatouille

This is a tasty side dish and makes a wonderful topping for fish, beef, and poultry dishes. Try it on baked potatoes!

Serves 4 (1½ cups = 1 serving)

      4 tablespoons olive oil
      1 onion, coarsely chopped
      1 green bell pepper, seeded, cut into 1-inch
         pieces
      1 eggplant, unpeeled, cut into 1-inch cubes
      2 zucchini, cut into ¼-inch rounds
      3 tomatoes, peeled, seeded, and chopped
      ½ teaspoon salt (optional)
      2 teaspoons chopped fresh basil or ½ teaspoon
         dried basil
      ½ teaspoon dried oregano
      2 garlic cloves, minced

In a large covered saucepan, sauté onion and green pepper in olive oil until lightly browned. Add eggplant and zucchini. Cook until tender. Add tomatoes, salt (optional), basil, and oregano. Cover and cook over low heat, stirring occasionally, 35 to 40 minutes. Add garlic and cook uncovered for 10 minutes.

Garlic Roasted Peppers and Anchovies

Serve as antipasto, salad, or vegetable. For those on a low-sodium diet, omit the anchovies.

Serves 4 (½ cup = 1 serving)

4 large bell peppers, halved, seeds and
   membranes removed (preferably a
   combination of green, red, and yellow)
1 head of garlic
1 tablespoon olive oil
¼ cup coarsely chopped fresh parsley
1 2-ounce can anchovy fillets, well drained and
   rinsed to remove extra salt

Preheat broiler. Roast peppers on baking sheet under open broiler, turning every few minutes until skin has browned. Remove peppers and put them in a brown paper bag to rest for at least 15 minutes. Peel skin and cut into long thin strips. Dry thoroughly on paper towels.

Separate garlic into cloves and place in boiling water for 15 minutes. Cool and remove skins. Place garlic, olive oil, parsley, and anchovies in a blender. Blend to make a paste. Toss paste with peppers and refrigerate 1 hour or longer before serving.

Minted Carrots and Snow Peas

A pleasing twist to an old favorite.

Serves 4 (½ cup = 1 serving)

6 carrots, cut into thin strips
1 teaspoon butter
¼ pound snow peas (Chinese pea pods), strings
   removed from both sides
1 teaspoon chopped fresh mint

Sauté carrots in butter 7 to 10 minutes. Add snow peas and cook an additional 1 to 2 minutes. Remove from heat. Stir in mint and serve.

Coleslaw with Anise, Caraway, and Poppy Seeds

A delicious coleslaw without mayonnaise.

Serves 4 (1 cup = 1 serving)

1 small head green cabbage, shredded
2 carrots, grated
½ cup nonfat plain yogurt
¼ teaspoon anise seeds
¼ teaspoon poppy seeds
¼ teaspoon caraway seeds
¼ teaspoon dry mustard
2 tablespoons fresh lemon juice

Place cabbage and carrots in mixing bowl. Combine yogurt, all the seeds, mustard, and lemon juice. Toss cabbage and carrots with yogurt mixture to cover thoroughly. Serve chilled.

SWEET DELIGHTS

New and exotic varieties of fruit are finding their way into mainstream markets, along with their vegetable cousins. Fiber-packed fruits are high in vitamins and minerals but low in sodium. They can be enjoyed as hot or cold cereal toppings, whether fresh or dried, and as low-calorie snacks between meals. Vary your fruit intake by enjoying the mildly tart taste of fresh kiwi, or try a plump persimmon cut in half and eaten like a melon. Fresh fruits can be frozen for several hours and then pureed into sugar-free sorbets. Bananas, berries, and peaches are tasty sorbet favorites. Succulent papaya, pineapple, guava, and mango are especially high in digestive enzymes and can help a sensitive digestive tract when eaten fully ripe. Enjoy fruit as the perfect snack all by itself, because its nutritional value is best utilized for digestion when not combined with other foods. This is also true for the fruit-based puddings and gelatins presented in this section.

If you are following the 21 Day Master Menu Plan, remember that Sweet Delights can be enjoyed as one of the 1–3 daily fruit servings after the three-week period.

Baked Apple with Raisins, Cinnamon, and Nutmeg

Baked apples provide a good fruit variation for breakfast or any time of day.

Serves 4 (1 apple = 1 serving)

    4 cooking apples, such as MacIntosh or Granny
      Smith, cored and pared
    1 tablespoon unsweetened apple juice
    2 tablespoons loose raisins
    1 teaspoon ground cinnamon
    ¼ teaspoon grated nutmeg

Preheat oven to 350°. Place apples and apple juice in baking dish. Fill centers with mixture of raisins, cinnamon, and nutmeg. Cover and bake for 45 minutes.

Vanilla Pears

Fresh peaches, plums, or nectarines can be substituted for pears when in season.

Serves 4 (2 pear halves = 1 serving)

    4 pears, cored, peeled, and halved
    1 tablespoon water
    1 teaspoon allspice
    12 drops vanilla extract

Preheat oven to 325°. Place pears and water in baking dish. Sprinkle with allspice and drizzle each pear half with 3 drops of vanilla extract. Cover and bake for about 20 minutes.

Old-Fashioned Applesauce

This is delicious served warm or chilled.

Serves 4 (½ cup = 1 serving)

    4 cooking apples, peeled, cored, and chopped
    2 tablespoons unsweetened apple juice

2 tablespoons honey
¼ teaspoon ground cinnamon
⅛ teaspoon grated nutmeg

In a saucepan, cook apples in apple juice over low to medium heat about 12 to 15 minutes. Cool slightly. Place in blender with honey, cinnamon, and nutmeg. Blend until smooth.

Rhubarb Sauce

Rhubarb, like applesauce, is good warm or chilled.

Serves 4 (½ cup = 1 serving)

1 pound rhubarb, chopped
1 tablespoon water
4 tablespoons honey
½ teaspoon cinnamon

In a saucepan, cook rhubarb in water over low to medium heat 10 to 15 minutes. Blend in honey and cinnamon.

The Magic Muffin

This muffin represents dietary magic because the oat bran component is a powerful cholesterol tamer.

Serves 8 (1 muffin = 1 serving)

2 teaspoons butter
1 cup + 2 tablespoons oat bran
1½ teaspoons baking powder
1 teaspoon ground cinnamon
¼ teaspoon salt (optional)
1 tablespoon chopped almonds
¼ cup + 2 tablespoons nonfat milk
1 egg, beaten
2 tablespoons honey
1 apple, cored and chopped

Preheat oven to 425°. Butter 8 muffin cups. Mix oat bran, baking powder, cinnamon, and salt (optional) in a bowl. Stir in almonds. In a separate bowl combine milk, egg, honey, and chopped apple. Make a well in dry ingredients and add milk mixture. Stir just until moistened. Spoon into prepared muffin cups. Bake for 15 minutes.

NOUVELLE PUDDINGS

Coconut Rum Pudding

Nutritious and delicious.

Serves 4 (½ cup = 1 serving)

    2 cups nonfat milk
    ⅛ teaspoon salt (optional)
    3 tablespoons arrowroot
    4 tablespoons honey
    1 egg, beaten
    ½ teaspoon coconut extract
    ½ teaspoon rum extract

In a saucepan, heat 1½ cups milk and salt (optional) at low to medium heat. Dissolve arrowroot in remaining ½ cup milk. Add arrowroot and milk to already heated milk and bring to gentle boil, stirring constantly as nonfat milk scorches easily. Reduce heat, add honey, and mix thoroughly. Add 1 cup of hot pudding mixture to egg in mixing bowl, stirring enough to heat egg but not cook it. Return to saucepan, stirring constantly to thoroughly mix all ingredients. Return to boil, still stirring constantly. Remove from heat. Add flavor extracts. Cool 20 minutes before refrigeration. Serve chilled.

Maple Pudding

An easy variation on the pudding theme.

Serves 4 (½ cup = 1 serving)

Follow recipe for Coconut Rum Pudding. Substitute 5 tablespoons maple syrup and ½ teaspoon pure maple flavoring for the coconut and rum extracts.

Fruit Compote Pudding

Another healthful variation to please a sweet tooth.

Serves 4 (½ cup = 1 serving)

Follow recipe for Coconut Rum Pudding. Mix ½ cup mixed sun-dried fruit (figs, dates, apricots) into pudding after removing from heat.

Tapioca Pudding

Who doesn't like tapioca pudding?

Serves 4 (½ cup = 1 serving)

    3 tablespoons granulated tapioca
    1½ cups nonfat milk
    ⅛ teaspoon salt (optional)
    3 tablespoons honey
    1 egg, beaten
    1 teaspoon vanilla extract

In a saucepan, heat tapioca, milk, and salt (optional) over low heat. Bring to a slow boil and cook uncovered for 5 minutes, stirring frequently. Reduce heat. Add honey and blend thoroughly. Pour some of the hot mixture into the egg in a mixing bowl, stirring enough to heat egg but not cook it. Return mixture to saucepan, stirring frequently, and bring to gentle boil. Simmer 3 minutes over low heat. Remove from heat and add vanilla extract. Cool 20 minutes before refrigerating. Serve chilled.

FRUIT GELATINS

Cherry Gelatin

Any unsweetened fruit juice can be used in this basic gelatin recipe. Health food stores carry many unusual

combinations of unsweetened fruit juice, such as papaya, apple-boysenberry, and apple-strawberry.

Serves 4 ($\frac{1}{2}$ cup = 1 serving)

    2 cups unsweetened cherry juice
    2 tablespoons agar-agar

Combine juice and agar-agar in saucepan. Boil for 30
seconds. Cool 20 minutes and refrigerate until set (about
2 hours). Serve chilled.

Piña Colada Gelatin

Serves 4 ($\frac{1}{2}$ cup = 1 serving)

Follow recipe for Cherry Gelatin, substituting unsweetened pineapple-coconut juice for cherry juice.

Pomegranate Gelatin

Serves 4 ($\frac{1}{2}$ cup = 1 serving)

Follow recipe for Cherry Gelatin, substituting pomegranate juice for cherry juice.

Carob Gelatin

It may not be chocolate pudding, but close enough.

Serves 4 ($\frac{1}{2}$ cup = 1 serving)

    $\frac{2}{3}$ cup Carob Dream dessert topping (from
       health food store)
    $1\frac{1}{3}$ cups water
    2 tablespoons agar-agar

Mix all ingredients in a saucepan and boil for 30 seconds. Cool 20 minutes and refrigerate until set (about 2
hours). Serve chilled.

FRESH FRUIT SORBETS

Blueberry Banana

This sorbet stands well on its own as an alternative to ice cream.

Serves 4 (½ cup = 1 serving)

> 1¾ cups blueberries (fresh or frozen)
> 2 bananas, sliced
> 1 tablespoon honey
> ½ teaspoon fresh lemon juice

Place all ingredients in food processor or blender and blend until smooth. Place in plastic container and freeze at least 2 hours. Take out partially frozen fruit and stir well to break up ice crystals. Return to freezer to completely freeze. Let fruit sorbet stand 15 minutes at room temperature before serving.

Ginger Pear Sorbet

A spicy fruit flavor to satisfy your taste buds.

Serves 4 (½ cup = 1 serving)

> 4 pears, peeled, cored, and cubed
> ¼ teaspoon powdered ginger
> 1 tablespoon honey
> ½ teaspoon fresh lemon juice

Place all ingredients in food processor or blender and blend until smooth. Freeze in plastic container for 2 hours. Take out partially frozen fruit and stir well to break up ice crystals. Return to freezer and freeze completely. Let stand at room temperature 15 minutes before serving.

Grain Creations

Whole-grain cereals are naturally high sources of fiber, minerals, and B vitamins. Their high complex-carbohydrate content sustains blood sugar levels because of the slow release of energy. The basic recipe for most grains is easy to remember: 2 cups of grain to 1 cup of water. Millet, barley, and wild rice require 3 cups of water, and corn meal needs 4 cups. The grain is added to the boiling water and simmered over low heat for about 30 to 40 minutes. Low, slow cooking temperatures do not destroy the minerals and vitamins that are vulnerable to the effects of high temperatures.

A tiny grain seed called amaranth is a fairly new addition to store shelves. It was widely used by the Aztecs in Mexico hundreds of years ago and was revered as a magical, mystical grain. Amaranth is one of the highest protein grains and is a good source of lysine, an essential amino acid lacking in most other grains. Amaranth can be used alone as a cereal or added to the batter of breads and baked goods. Added to popcorn, it can also be popped, although the grain does not expand.

Another exotic high-protein grain is quinoa. Reputed to be as high or higher in protein value than amaranth, quinoa is an abundant source of the amino acids methionine and cystine as well as lysine. Known as the "mother grain" of the Incas, quinoa is low in gluten and makes a nutritious substitute for wheat-sensitive individuals.

For cold winter mornings, I suggest either rye or buckwheat groats (or kasha). These hearty cereals are good for the circulation and will keep you warm. In hot weather you can choose from any of the other varieties eaten cold, already prepared.

Food Equivalents

Your kitchen is your personal health laboratory. The following exchange lists are designed for your culinary creativity. You can substitute, mix, or match the food choices to fit your needs and tastes. Each food portion is interchangeable with all others listed in the same group because, in the portions given, they provide the same kinds of nutrients.

Brand names are generally not specified in this section. Refer to "Stocking and Storing the Staples" (p. 141) for preferred brands.

The Essential and Healthy Fats

A combined total of 2 tablespoons can be chosen from among the following recommended fat equivalents. The 2 tablespoon amount is the daily quantity necessary to meet nutritional requirements and appetite satisfaction. The higher amount of essential fatty acids contained in expeller-pressed safflower, sunflower, corn, and soy especially activate your fat burner to convert calories into heat rather than store them as fat for effective and lasting weight loss.

Each food source is broken down to equal the equivalent of 1 tablespoon of oil, so that you have the option to vary your beneficial fat intake from a number of delicious sources.

Crude or unrefined oils (expeller-pressed)	1 tablespoon
Avocado	½ small
Nuts (raw or home-toasted)	15 small
Seeds (raw or home-toasted)	1½ teaspoons
Sesame seed butter	1 tablespoon
Mayonnaise (commercially made from expeller-pressed oil or homemade with expeller-pressed oil)	1 tablespoon

Protein

Include a total of 6 to 8 ounces daily from any combination of the following protein sources. Each food source is broken down to equal the equivalent of 1 ounce of fish, poultry, or lean beef. Limit egg intake to 4 to 6 per week. It is best to spread out protein foods throughout the day, dividing them between breakfast, lunch, and dinner.

Cheese	¼ cup
Egg	1
Fish and seafood	
Salmon, halibut, perch, sole:	1 ounce
Oysters, clams, shrimp, scallops:	5 small
Anchovies (well rinsed):	9 fillets
Sardines:	3 medium
Canned Salmon, tuna, crab:	¼ cup
Poultry and beef	
Turkey, chicken, beef, veal, lamb:	1 ounce
Tofu	1 ounce

Vegetables

Include a daily total of 4 or more servings from the list below. Each serving equals ½ cup (4 ounces). Celery, cucumbers, endive, escarole, lettuce, radishes, and assorted sprouts are especially desirable for meal planning and snacking because of their low-calorie content and should be counted as "freebies."

Artichoke (1 small whole)	Endive
Bamboo shoots	Escarole
Beans, green or yellow	Greens: beets, chard, kale,
Beets	collard, dandelion,
Broccoli	mustard, spinach,
Brussels sprouts	turnip, radicchio,
Cabbage	arugula, mache,
Carrots (1 medium)	broccoli rabe
Cauliflower	Jicama
Celery	Jerusalem artichoke
Chicory	(sunchoke)
Chilies: green or red	Mushrooms
Chinese cabbage	Okra
Cucumbers	Onions
Eggplant	Peppers: green or red

Radishes: red or Daikon
Rutabaga
Sauerkraut
Seaweed: nori and kelp
Sprouts: mung bean,
    adzuki, alfalfa, clover,
    radish
Squash: summer,
    spaghetti, chayote

Snow peas
Tomatoes
Tomato juice
Turnips
Vegetable juice cocktail
Water chestnuts (4)
Watercress
Zucchini

Note: Herbs—parsley, cilantro, basil, mint, oregano, rosemary, dill, tarragon, marjoram, etc.—can be used freely.

Fruits

These fruits are the recommended snacks to be enjoyed between meals. Eat a maximum of 3 fruits daily.

Apple	1 small (2-inch diameter)
Apple butter (sugar free)	2 tablespoons
Apple juice or cider	1/3 cup
Applesauce (unsweetened)	1/2 cup
Apricots (fresh)	2 medium
Apricots (dried)	4 halves
Banana	1/2 small
Berries: boysenberries, blackberries, blueberries, raspberries	1/2 cup
Cantaloupe	1/4 (6-inch diameter)
Cherries	10 large
Dates	2
Figs (fresh)	1 large
Figs (dried)	1 small
Fruit cocktail (in its juice)	1/2 cup
Fruit preserves & spreads (sugar free)	2 tablespoons
Grapefruit	1/2 small
Grapefruit juice	1/2 cup

Grapes	12
Grape juice	¼ cup
Honeydew melon	⅛ (7-inch diameter)
Mandarin oranges	¾ cup
Kiwi	1 medium
Mango	½ small
Nectarine	1 small
Orange	1 small
Orange juice	½ cup
Papaya	¾ cup
Peach	1 medium
Pear	1 small
Persimmon	1 medium
Pineapple	½ cup
Pineapple juice	⅓ cup
Plums	2 medium
Prunes	2 medium
Prune juice	¼ cup
Raisins	2 tablespoons
Strawberries	¾ cup
Tangerine	1 large
Watermelon	1 cup

Complex Carbohydrates

Include 2 OR MORE SERVINGS from the following variety on a daily basis. This is the group where servings can be added or subtracted, depending upon weight loss needs. Grain selections, particularly gluten-based cereals such as wheat, oats, rye, and barley should be kept to a minimum. The starchy vegetable group should be emphasized.

Starchy Vegetables:

Corn (on the cob)	1 (4″ long)
Corn (cooked)	⅓ cup
Parsnips	1 small
Peas (fresh)	¾ cup
Potatoes (sweet, yam)	¼ cup

Potatoes, white (baked or boiled)	1 small
Potatoes, white (mashed)	½ cup
Pumpkin	¾ cup
Rutabaga	1 small
Squash (winter, acorn, butternut)	½ cup

Breads:

Bagel, whole wheat	½ small
Bread rye, pumpernickel, whole wheat	1 slice
Breadsticks	4 (7″ long)
Bun hamburger, hot dog	½
Croutons	½ cup
English muffin	½
English muffin	½
Pancakes	2 (3″ diam.)
Pita bread	½ of 6″ pocket
Rice cakes	2
Roll	1 (2″ diam.)
Tortilla	1 (6″ diam.)

Cereals and Grains:

Barley (cooked)	½ cup
Bran flakes	½ cup
Bran (unprocessed rice or wheat)	⅓ cup
Buckwheat groats (kasha) (cooked)	⅓ cup
Cream of rice (cooked)	½ cup
Grapenuts	¼ cup
Grits (cooked)	½ cup
Millet (cooked)	½ cup
Oatmeal	½ cup
Popcorn	3 cups
Puffed rice, wheat, millet & oats	1½ cups

Rice (brown, cooked)	⅓ cup
Rice (wild, cooked)	½ cup
Shredded wheat biscuit	1 large
Wheatena (cooked)	½ cup
Wheat germ	1 oz. or 3 Tbsp.

Crackers:

Matzoh, whole wheat	½ (6″ × 4″)
Pretzels, whole grain	1 large
Rice Wafers, brown rice (Westbrae)	4
Rye crispbread crackers (Wasa)	1½ crackers
Wheat crackers, whole wheat (Ak-Mak)	4 crackers
(Health Valley)	13 crackers

Flours:

Arrowroot	2 Tbsp
Buckwheat	3 Tbsp
Cornmeal	3 Tbsp
Cornstarch	2 Tbsp
Potato flour	2½ Tbsp
Rice flour	3 Tbsp
Soya powder	3 Tbsp
Whole wheat	3 Tbsp

Legumes:

Beans, dried (cooked) lima, soy, navy, pinto, kidney, garbanzos, black	½ cup
Beans, baked plain	½ cup
Lentils, dried (cooked)	½ cup
Peas, dried (cooked)	½ cup

Pasta

Noodles, macaroni, spaghetti (cooked)	½ cup

Noodles, rice (cooked)	½ cup
Noodles, whole wheat (cooked)	½ cup
Pasta, whole wheat (cooked)	½ cup

Dairy (optional)

The daily intake of 2 servings of cow's milk, nonfat dairy products, or goat's milk products from the following alternatives is up to you. Remember, the label should read "0 grams fat" to qualify as a healthy fat cow's milk dairy product. Many who cannot tolerate cow's milk do well with goat's milk, especially children.

Milk: nonfat cow's milk, goat's milk	1 cup
Yogurt: nonfat cow's milk, plain; goat's milk yogurt, plain	1 cup 1 cup
Soya powder (substitute for milk)	3 tablespoons

Note: If you can find pasteurized, nonhomogenized cow's milk, you can use it to replace both the nonfat and the goat's milk servings cup for cup. Just pour off the cream and give it to your grateful friends.

Ten Transitional Tips

The following dietary suggestions will assist you in changing to a healthier eating plan:

• One tablespoon of freshly ground flaxseed (kept in fridge or freezer) can be added to cereal right before serving time. It's a great natural laxative for both young and old.

• Use Worcestershire sauce to replace soy sauce. Worcestershire contains 55 mg. of sodium per tablespoon, as compared to 1000 mg. of sodium per tablespoon in soy sauce. The flavor is great with sauces, meatloaf, and even on vegetables.

• To replace cream and whole milk in soups and sauces, substitute arrowroot and/or instant mashed potatoes from health food store.

• Pureed vegetables such as winter squash, broccoli, carrots, sweet potatoes, and green peas are great for side dishes drizzled with a drop of virgin olive oil.

• Ground turkey can replace ground beef in loaves.

• For added fat-fighting fiber, mix 1 tablespoon oat bran in your hot cereal.

• Cranberry sauce is a low sodium, virtually fat-free replacement for heavy gravies on meat, fish, and poultry.

• Grated orange peel or lemon rind with ground nutmeg is a zesty cooking pickup. Add to fish or chicken before broiling and to squash before baking.

• Horseradish (either prepared or powdered) can be added to nonfat yogurt as a quick and easy dip, or sauce for fish and vegetables. The recipe is 1 tablespoon horseradish to 1 cup nonfat yogurt.

• For hard-core hamburger lovers, try 1 teaspoon of Angostura Bitters to 1 pound lean ground beef to substitute for bacon, cheese, and mayonnaise.

19

SPICES AND HERBS OF LIFE

*The earth yields her seed, her vegetables, her fruit and
her greens; use as the Creator provided them.*
—ANN WIGMORE, raw foods pioneer

Folk medicine for centuries touted the healing effects of
certain herbs and spices. Herbs are especially rich in the
minerals manganese, potassium, and iron. Dill, fennel,
mint, and savory are all reputed to aid digestion, while
rosemary was prized in Shakespeare's time to be good
for the memory, sage tea was considered a strongly medicinal spring tonic, and thyme was revered as a medie-
val symbol of courage. Bay leaves have always been used
to keep bugs out of the cupboard and out of flour, and
oil of cloves can relieve a toothache.

Herbal Magic

Many modern medicines have their origins in herbs
(such as digitalis from the foxglove plant and aspirin
from willow bark). Valium, the most widely prescribed
tranquilizer, is based on the herb valerian root. Capsules
of powdered ginger are a modern day preventive against
motion sickness. Cardamom is revered as an aphrodis-
iac in the Middle East. The antioxidant properties of
rosemary are now being extracted for use as natural
food preservatives.

It is the volatile oil in each herb that contains much of the herb's health-enhancing qualities. To release the volatile oil, use a mortar and pestle or a small grinder. To preserve the oil, store in a tightly sealed opaque container in a cool place away from the stove, oven, or dishwasher. You can protect ground herbs and spices from the ravages of heat, air, and light in these ways.

Essential oils can be used instead of dried herbs and spices. They have a longer shelf life than their herb and spice counterparts and blend better with other recipe ingredients. One teaspoon of dried herb or spice is equal to two drops of the essential oil. While there are many oils that can be used safely in cooking, such as peppermint, anise, rosemary, lemon, and lime, not all oils are suitable for consumption.

Seasoning Savvy

Here are some of my flavoring favorites that add spice to your palate without added salt, sugar, or damaged fats. Wines and liqueurs are good flavor boosters because the alcohol and calories are burned off in cooking, while the flavor remains. The flavorful skins of lemons, limes, and oranges (with the white membrane detached) add zing to a number of foods. These "zests," like herbs, spices, wines, and liqueurs, are also piquant cooking essences.

Spices are not only tasty, they can also help you burn more calories and control blood sugar levels. Cayenne pepper, ginger, and mustard can all increase metabolism. Did you know that a mere teaspoon of dried mustard has a 25 percent metabolic-raising effect up to three hours after ingestion?

Sugar cravings can be deliciously relieved with cinnamon, cloves, and bay leaves.

FOOD	FLAVOR FIXER
FISH	Basil, dillweed, ginger, garlic, fennel, chervil, onions, lemon zest, capers, saffron, Pernod, dry sherry

MEAT

Beef	Thyme, cumin, horseradish, basil, clove, garlic, curry, cardamom, red wine
Lamb	Rosemary, mint, cinnamon, garlic, allspice, curry
Poultry	Tarragon, rosemary, curry, paprika, lemon zest, garlic, mustard, horseradish, sage, thyme, lime zest, vodka, tequila

EGGS — Black pepper, nutmeg, white wine, parsley, chervil

BEANS — Thyme, coriander, sage, garlic, shallots, chives, curry, savory, cumin, turmeric, beer

SOUPS — Bay leaf, dill, parsley, onions, celery seed, sherry

VEGETABLES

Asparagus	Tarragon, parsley, mustard seed, lemon zest
Beets	Dill, cloves, savory, garlic, ginger, bay leaf
Broccoli	Mustard seed, onion, garlic, tarragon
Brussels sprouts	Basil, sage, thyme, garlic, caraway seed
Cabbage	Caraway seed, mint, nutmeg, savory, ginger, gin, allspice
Carrots	Allspice, dill, marjoram, bay leaf, fennel, ginger, Pernod
Cauliflower	Celery seed, mace, caraway seed, tarragon, cumin
Cucumber	Basil, dill, mint
Eggplant	Oregano, marjoram
Greens	Chives, dill, tarragon, basil
Onions	Thyme, nutmeg, oregano, sage
Peas	Rosemary, savory, poppy seed, mint
Potatoes	Chives, bay leaf, thyme, caraway seed
Spinach	Basil, mace, nutmeg, marjoram
Squash	Cloves, fennel, ginger, nutmeg
Sweet potatoes	Cardamom, cinnamon, cloves, allspice

| Tomatoes | Basil, celery seed, sesame seed, capers, Pernod, dry Madeira |
| | *Note:* Fennel and anise seed give a sausage flavor to tomato sauce |

FRUITS

Apples	Allspice, cinnamon, nutmeg, coriander, ginger
Pears	Cardamom, vanilla extract, champagne
Bananas	All wines, brandy, rum
Compote	All wines, brandy, rum
Dried fruit mixtures	Fruit brandies
Grapefruit	Bourbon (*Note:* A drop of olive oil brushed on a grapefruit, then broiled, sweetens it considerably. Bitters are also very good on grapefruit.)

Spice It Up

If you like experimenting with different combinations of flavors, here are some suggestions to get started.

Oriental blends on fish and chicken (ginger, cinnamon, anise, nutmeg, and cloves)

Italian blends on steamed vegetables (oregano, marjoram, thyme, savory, basil, and rosemary)

Indian blends on grains and beans (cumin, dill, allspice, cardamom, and turmeric)

Mexican blends on egg dishes (chili pepper, garlic powder, and cumin)

Pumpkin Pie spice on oatmeal or squash (cinnamon, ginger, allspice, and nutmeg)

Some Like It Hot

Cajun seasonings are now available in seven varieties from Paul Prudhommes's Cajun Magic spices. Call 1-800-654-6017 for the nearest outlet or to order direct.

20

EATING OUT SMART

*Gaining health without maintaining it is like winning the war
but losing the peace.*
—Anonymous

Whether you are on land, in the air, or traveling the high
seas, following the *Beyond Pritikin* Diet can be a satisfying proposition. Fish and fiber-rich foods, like beans,
grains, vegetables, salads, and fruit are your mainstays,
and these can be found almost everywhere. Food selection outside the home has become fun and convenient
due to the popularity of salad bars and the addition of
lighter entrees for the calorie conscious in most restaurants across the country.

The golden rule is simple: Order mainly foods containing the essential or healthy fats. Best bets are all
kinds of fish and shellfish, grilled, broiled, and poached
or baked in wine and seasoned with garlic and onions.
Fresh salads, steamed vegetables, corn on the cob, and
plain baked potatoes (you can add a dot of butter for
flavor) are wise food choices. Ask for fruit for dessert or
eat it as a snack between meals. Olive oil is probably the
only available healthful fat cooking and salad oil you will
be able to order, but go easy with the olive oil, about 1
tablespoon per meal to be exact. You can truly enjoy this

taste treat guilt-free because it is a heart-healthy fat choice.

Remember that the undesirable hidden fats, salts, and sugars abound in sauces and dressings. Choose simple dishes and request *all* sauces on the side. In this way you have more control over flavor and the bad fats. Side orders of sliced onions or chives are usually available at most restaurants and are an easy source of flavor. A small dab of butter can add a grateful touch to otherwise tasteless cooked vegetables.

Remember that tuna, chicken, and egg salad usually contain too much mayonnaise and so should be avoided on a daily basis. Actually, mayonnaise is a processed food, containing heat-treated and partially hydrogenated oil, in the form of partially hydrogenated soybean oil. Wherever possible, substitute small amounts of mustard or yogurt for mayonnaise.

Where's the Beef?

In standard restaurants when fish is not available or you feel like a change, turkey, chicken, and lean ground beef are good alternatives. Yes, lean beef. Eaten in moderation, about twice a week, beef has a respectable place on the menu. There are several trace minerals such as copper, iron, zinc, and manganese that red meat provides and that cannot be found in such high amounts in other foods. Lean roast beef is a viable choice. Chef's salads (without the ham), Greek, and Niçoise are also smart selections.

Oatmeal and poached or soft-, medium-, and hard-cooked eggs are easily obtainable for breakfast in most places. A good luncheon or dinner meal might consist of a hearty soup such as minestrone, lentil, mushroom, barley, or Manhattan clam chowder. Soups are great with a salad and a slice of whole-wheat or rye bread. You can skim off any excess fat in the soup by dropping in an ice cube and scooping the melted cube off the top along with the fat, which has been brought to the surface.

Small Plates

In some of the newer restaurants, creative diners can design their own meals by selecting appetizers and salads without main courses. Several fine eateries even offer the entire menu scaled down to appetizer-portion size often called tapas. This trend is a boon to Eating Out Smart because the wide variety of vegetables, light proteins, and salads fits the guidelines set by the Diet.

Beyond Pritikin Ethnic Eating

When Americans eat out, says a Gallup poll taken in 1985, they choose from American-style restaurants (56 percent), followed by Italian (14 percent), Chinese (12 percent), Mexican (8 percent), with French and Japanese last (at 2 percent). In each of these restaurants you can order safely and walk out feeling completely satisfied.

Italian Restaurants

For a change of pace at Italian restaurants, you might enjoy a pasta with pesto sauce (that delightful combination of basil, garlic, and olive oil with pine nuts). This is the place where you can make starch, in the form of pasta or beans, the focus of your meal. Remember your food combinations and do not combine wheat (the pasta dishes) with a meat or clam sauce. Meatless marinara or plain garlic and oil are good alternatives to the pesto sauce. Pasta primavera—pasta with vegetables—is an excellent choice. If pasta is not your thing, then order veal as your main entree. Veal marsala, piccata, and scallopini are delicious with a leafy green salad and sautéed vegetables.

Chinese Restaurants

First specify that your dishes be made without monosodium glutamate (MSG), sugar, salt, and soy sauce. Then inquire about the oil used in cooking. Many Chinese restaurants use peanut oil. If so, you are in luck. If not, then specify no oil along with the other omissions (MSG, sugar, and soy sauce). Assuming that peanut oil is used, choose chicken, shrimp, and flank steak dishes with steamed rice and vegetables, such as snow peas, water chestnuts, onion, broccoli, scallions, bamboo shoots, and Chinese cabbage (bok choy). Stir-fries with sprouts, vegetables, cellophane noodles (rice or mung bean noodles) and small amounts of chicken, beef, tofu, or seafood are tasty choices. Buddha's Delight (a mixed vegetable dish) is always a winner. The fortune—without the cookie—is for dessert.

Mexican Restaurants

In the Mexican restaurants, black bean soup, gazpacho, and small amounts of guacamole laced with lots of fresh lemon or lime juice are tasty selections. Tortillas can be steamed instead of fried, and chili with or without the carne might also please your palate. Chicken with rice or shrimp with rice is a wise entree selection. Do avoid refried beans, which are usually made with lard.

French Restaurants

Choose "nouvelle cuisine," which is much lighter than the traditional French fare. Ordering food grilled, broiled, poached, or sautéed in wine such as a Bordelaise sauce is advisable. Watch out for those heavy cheese or cream sauces. Fish en papillote, a French favorite, is a delicious way to cook fish in its own juices.

Other Ethnic Choices

In Greek or Middle Eastern restaurants, hummus (garbanzo bean pâté with sesame butter, garlic, and lemon) and pita bread are usually available. Babaghanoush (eggplant pâté with sesame butter, garlic, and lemon) makes a great dip with vegetables. Tzatziki (yogurt and cucumber) is a good salad dressing. You can choose rice-based pilafs and tabbouleh (bulgur wheat, parsley, onion, tomato salad with olive oil and lemon). Salads that feature feta cheese (goat's cheese) are additional nutritious choices. Souvlaki (a combination of highly seasoned lamb and beef) is for those who like it hot, otherwise shish kabob with meat and vegetables is for tamer souls.

In Indian restaurants, tandoori chicken and lamb are good choices. Yogurt sauces and vegetables cooked in ghee (clarified butter) are permissible in small amounts. The pilafs, biryanis, dals (legume containing dishes) are delicious. Curry seasonings are healthful for those who can take a little heat. The pappadums (lentil wafers) are great munchies *if* they are baked, not fried. The same goes for chapatis and nan (garlic or onion bread).

Safe Flying

Call ahead at least twenty-four hours in advance to arrange for special food. Some airlines have diet menus approved by the American Heart Association. Others are also very accommodating for special dietary needs. You can usually order a cold seafood plate no matter which airline you fly, and be reasonably satisfied with what you get.

Cruising Cuisine

Like the airlines, the cruise lines also try to fulfill dietary requests made with a twenty-four-hour lead time. Leaner luncheon and dinner entrees that meet the dietary guidelines of the American Heart Association are becoming common fare among the more popular cruise lines.

Managing Margarine

The American Heart Association itself sponsors restaurants in every city of America that comply with their
low-fat, low-cholesterol, low-sodium dietary recommendations. Keep in mind, however, that low fat, low cholesterol does not mean good fat, because margarine is still
on the A.H.A. approved list. Request *no margarine* on any
of your foods, whatever you order. Low-fat, low-cholesterol menus are a good start for most commercial eateries. Just be careful and avoid the margarine!

Major cities such as Chicago, Baltimore, Palm Beach,
San Francisco, and Los Angeles are active participants in
the A.H.A. restaurant program. Many hotel chains also
participate. On the West Coast and the East Coast you
can usually find restaurants that serve A.H.A.-approved
meals. The menu will note A.H.A. approval.

APPENDIX

NUTRITION EDUCATION RESOURCES

Everyone should be his own physician.
We ought to assist, not force nature.
—VOLTAIRE

We all need good self-care educational resources. Here are some of my favorites:

> **American Academy of Nutrition**
> 3408 Sausalito
> Corona del Mar, CA 92625-1638
> (800) 290-4226

The American Academy of Nutrition offers nutritional education courses through home study. It is the only nutrition home-study school in the world accredited by the Accreditation Commission of the Distance Education and Training Council, which is the only U.S. Department of Education–listed agency accrediting home-study schools. The Academy is also approved as a continuing education provider for many groups, including nurses and the American College of Sports Medicine, and is approved by the U.S. Department of Defense for military tuition assistance. In addition, its courses are recognized for college credit. As Director of Continuing Education for the American Academy of Nutrition, I highly recommend the nutrition courses for anyone who wishes to increase his or her knowledge in a variety of health areas.

Some of the courses include:

- Vegetarian Nutrition
- Nutrition Counseling
- Sports Nutrition
- Women's Health Issues

Bio/Tech News
Box 30568
Parkrose Center
Portland, OR 97230
(206) 254-5876

Bio/Tech News is a state-of-the-art newsletter that focuses on "inside information on important innovations in BioScience and Technology." Topics such as parasites, colloidal silver, pots and pans, and even bowel toxemia and digestive enzymes are dealt with in a very timely manner.

Citizens for Health
P.O. Box 368
Tacoma, WA 98401
(206) 922-2457

This consumer-oriented group is dedicated to keeping you informed about the latest government regulations affecting health-care options. Citizens for Health has an immediate fax network and a quarterly newsletter. You can join for $20, benefactors for $75, and founders for $250. Each of these rates entitles you to different benefits.

Natural Lifestyling
P.O. Box 21070
Albuquerque, NM 87154
(505) 821-7186

This monthly magazine is a very informative resource guide for holistic health and natural living. I have been a featured writer for many years, so you may be interested in back issues.

A one-year subscription (twelve issues) is $18; back issues are $2 each.

Townsend Letter for Doctors
911 Tyler Street
Port Townsend, WA 98368-6541
(206) 385-6021

The *Townsend Letter* is a self-proclaimed "informal letter magazine for doctors communicating with doctors." It focuses on current nutritional issues, legislation, and research with a preventive and holistic slant. The *Townsend Letter* is published monthly.

The Price-Pottenger Nutrition Foundation
P.O. Box 2614
La Mesa, CA 91943-2614
(619) 574-7763

Now you can locate a nutrition-oriented health-care professional who can help you personally apply the nutritional information found in this book. Simply send a $6.00 donation to the address above. Please indicate the state for which you are requesting a referral listing. Contact PPNF for:

- Referrals to nutrition-oriented health-care professionals
- Catalog of books, audio- and videotapes, slides, etc.
- Ecology, nutrition, and organic farming resources
- Membership information
- Quarterly *PPNF Journal* and *Eco-Nutritional News*

The Price-Pottenger Nutrition Foundation is a nonprofit, tax-exempt educational organization dedicated to the promotion of enhanced health through awareness of ecology, lifestyle, and healthy food production for sound nutrition. At its core are the landmark works of Drs. Weston A. Price and Francis M. Pottenger, Jr., pioneers in modern research.

Organic Food Business News
Hotline Printing and Publishing
P.O. Box 161132
Altamonte Springs, FL 32716
(407) 628-1377

Organic Food Business News is a monthly international news-letter that tracks the latest financial trends, mergers, and new companies, and provides special reports on segments of the industry.

Allergy Hotline
Hotline Printing and Publishing
P.O. Box 161132
Altamonte Springs, FL 32716
(407) 628-1377

Allergy Hotline is a monthly newsletter distributed to physicians and allergy patients and features the latest news, research, homeopathic remedies, and alternative diets.

FDA Hotline
Hotline Printing and Publishing
P.O. Box 161132
Altamonte Springs, FL 32716
(407) 628-1377

FDA Hotline is a monthly newsletter for dietary and vitamin-supplement companies as well as homeopathic physicians that tracks legislation, enforcement actions, raids, and court filings.

Biosocial Publications International
P.O. Box 1174
Tacoma, WA 98401

This organization provides two unusual nutrition-related journals. *The International Journal of Biosocial Research*, available semiannually, presents original studies and articles on how nutrition, biochemistry, and environment relate to human behavior. *The International Nutrition Review* is a quarterly publication that reports on current health research from around the world. The organization also has a catalog of carefully selected nutrition books that are relevant to many areas of nutritional science.

The Felix Letter
Clara Felix
P.O. Box 7094
Berkeley, CA 94707

The Felix Letter is a well researched, highly documented newsletter from nutritionist Clara Felix. Several issues deal with the importance of oils in the American diet. Ms. Felix provides a special slant, as a professional nutritionist, on many contemporary issues ranging from elixirs of youth to good versus bad prostaglandins to hormone replacement. Her commentary on nutrition is laced with cartoons, photos, and original illustrations. She has published almost 100 issues to date—every one a gem.

For specialty food products (such as Celtic Salt, Balance Bars, Capri Mineral Whey coffee substitute), water filters, and my books:

Uni Key Health Systems
P.O. Box 7168
Bozeman, MT 59771
(800) 888-4353

REFERENCES

Ames, B. "Dietary Carcinogens & Anti-Carcinogens": Oxygen Radicals and Degenerative Disease." *Science* 221 (1980): 1245.

Anderson, J., et al. "Oat bran intake selectively lowers serum low density lipoprotein cholesterol concentrations of hypercholesterolemic men." *American Journal of Clinical Nutrition* 34 (1981): 824.

———. "Hypocholesterolemic effects of oat bran or bean intake for hypercholesterolemic men." *American Journal of Clinical Nutrition* 40 (1984): 1146.

Anderson, R. A., and A. S. Kozlosky. "Chromium intake, absorption and excretion of subjects consuming self-selected diets." *American Journal of Clinical Nutrition* 41 (1985): 1177–83.

Ascherio, A., et al. "Trans fatty intake and risk of myocardial infarction." *Circulation* 89 (January 1994): 94–101.

Beare-Rogers, J., et al. "The linoleic acid and trans fatty acids of margarines." *American Journal of Clinical Nutrition* 32 (1979): 1805.

Bieler, Henry, M.D. *Food Is Your Best Medicine.* (New York: Ballantine Books, 1984.)

"Biological Rhythms in Psychiatry and Medicine." National Institute of Mental Health. National Clearinghouse for Mental Health Information, pp. 120–32.

BioSyn Position Paper. "The GLA and ALA Connection." BioSyn, Marblehead, MA 01945.

Bland, Jeffrey, Ph.D. *Your Health Under Siege.* (Brattleboro, VT: The Stephen Green Press, 1981.)

Booyens, J., et al. "The role of unnatural dietary trans and cis unsaturated fatty acids in the epidemiology of coronary artery disease." *Medical Hypothesis* 25 (1988): 175–82.

Bordia, A., et al. "Effect of the essential oils of garlic and onion on alimentary hyperlipidemia." *Atherosclerosis* 21 (1975): 15.

Brodeur, Paul. *The Zapping of America.* (New York: Norton, 1977.)

Brody, Liz. "Fat Phobia." *Shape,* March 1993: 104–7, 136–42.

Brown, M. "Fast Foods Are Hazardous to Your Health." *Science Digest,* April 1986: 31.

Budwig, Johanna, Dr. *Flax Oil as a True Aid Against Arthritis, Heart Infarction, Cancer and Other Diseases.* (Vancouver: Apple Publishing Co., 1992.)

Burkitt, D. "Some Neglected Leads to Cancer Causation." *Journal of the National Cancer Institute,* 47, no. 4 (1971): 913.

Burros, Marian. "Low-fat Diets: How Low to Go?" *New York Times,* January 12, 1994: C4+.

Cheraskin, Emanuel, M.D., D.M.D., and W. Ringsdorf, Jr., D.M.D., M.S., with Arline Brecher. *Psychodietetics.* (New York: Stein and Day, 1974.)

Cleave, T. *The Saccharine Disease.* (New Canaan, CT: Keats Publishing, 1974.)

Clement, Mark. *Aluminum: A Menace to Health.* (Sussex, England: Health Science Press, 1971.)

Clouatre, Dallas, Ph.D. *Anti-Fat Nutrients.* (San Francisco: Pax Publishing, 1993.)

Crapper, Dr., et al. "Essential fatty acid requirements in infancy." *American Journal of Clinical Nutrition* 31 (1978): 2181–85.

Crawford, M.A., et al. "Essential fatty acid requirements in infancy." *American Journal of Clinical Nutrition* 31 (1978): 2181–85.

Crayhon, Robert, M.S. *Nutrition Made Simple.* (New York: M. Evans & Co., Inc., 1995.)

Crook, William, M.D. *The Yeast Connection.* (Jackson, Tennessee: Professional Books, 1984.)

Dyerberg, J., and H. O. Bang. "Eicosapentaenoic acid and prevention of thrombosis and atherosclerosis?" *Lancet* 2 (1978): 117.

———. "Lipid metabolism, atherogenesis and haemostasis in

Eskimos; the role of the prostaglandin-3 family." *Haemostasis* 8 (1979): 227.

Elmer-Dewitt, Philip. "Fat Times." *Time*, January 19, 1995: 59–63.

Enig, Mary, Ph.D. *Trans Fatty Acids in the Food Supply: A Comprehensive Report Covering 60 Years of Research*. (Silver Spring, MD: Enig Associates, 1993.)

En-Trophy Institute Review 4 (March 6, 1980). "The Dietary Maginot Line." Community Nutrition Institute.

Erasmus, Udo. *Fats That Heal, Fats That Kill*. (Burnaby: Alive Books, 1993.)

Erickson, D. R., ed., et al. *Handbook of Soy Oil Processing and Utilization*. Third printing. (St. Louis, Missouri and Champaign, Illinois: American Soybean Association and American Oil Chemists' Society, 1985.)

Erlander, Stig, Ph.D. *Dr. Erlander's Pathway to Health*. (Altadena, CA: P.O. Box 106, Altadena, CA, 1980.)

Evans, G. W. "The effect of chromium picolinate on insulin controlled parameters in humans." *International Journal of Biosocial Medical Research* 11(2) (1989): 163–80.

Ezrin, Calvin, M.D., and Robert Kowalski. *The Endocrine Control Diet*. (New York: Harper & Row, 1990.)

"Facts About Food Poisoning" FDA Consumer Memo. Washington, DC: DHEW Publication No. (FDA) 74–2046 (April 1974).

Finnegan, John. *The Facts About Fats*. (Berkeley: First Celestial Arts Printing, 1993.)

Foster, D. "Insulin resistance—a secret killer?" *New England Journal of Medicine*, March 16, 1989, 733–734.

Freidman, Meyer. *Treating Type A Behavior and Your Heart*. (New York; Alfred A. Knopf, 1984.)

Gibson, R. A., and G. M. Kneebone. "Fatty acid composition of human colostrum and human breast milk." *American Journal of Clinical Nutrition* 34 (1981): 252–57.

Grundy, S. "Comparison of Monosaturated Fatty Acids and Carbohydrates for Lowering Plasma Cholesterol." *New England Journal of Medicine* 314, no. 12 (1986): 745.

Haflick, L. "On Those Magical Prostaglandins." *Executive Health* 16 (1980): 8.

Hall, Ross Hume. *Food For Nought*. (New York: Harper & Row, 1974.)

Health From the Sun Position Papers. "EPA Containing Marine Oils—a Consumer's Guide," "Evening Primrose Oil—a Guide for the Consumer," and "Technical Specifications of Edible Oils—a Consumer's Guide." Health from the Sun Products, Inc. Needham Heights, MA 02194.

Health Research. *The Story of Aluminum Poisoning*. Health Research, Mokelumne Hill, CA 95245.

Hepburn, F. N., et al. "Provisional tables on the content of omega-3 fatty acids and other fat components of selected foods." *Journal of the American Dietetic Association* 86 (1986): 788–93.

Himms, Hagen, J. "Thermogenesis in Brown Adipose Tissue as an Energy Buffer." *New England Journal of Medicine* 311 (1984): 1549.

Hirai, A., et al. "Eicosapentaenoic acid and platelet function in Japanese." *Lancet* 2 (1985): 1132.

Holman, R. T., ed. *Progress in Lipid Research*. Vol. 20. (New York: Pergamon Press, 1982.)

———, et al. "Effects of trans fatty acid isomers upon essential fatty acid deficiency in rats." *Proceedings of the Society for Experimental Biology and Medicine* 93 (1956): 175–79.

———, et al. *Dietary Fats and Health*. E. G. Perkins and W. J. Visek, eds. (Champaign, IL: American Oil Chemists Society Press, 1983.)

Horrobin, David F., M.D., Ph.D. *Clinical Uses of Essential Fatty Acids*. (Montreal-London: Eden Press, 1982.)

———, et al. "The nutritional regulation of T-lymphocyte function." *Medical Hypothesis* 5 (1979): 969.

———. "Schizophrenia: the role of abnormal essential fatty acid and prostaglandin metabolism." Rev. *Drug Metabolism Drug Interaction* 4 (1983): 339.

———. "The regulation of prostaglandin biosynthesis by the manipulation of essential fatty acid metabolism." Rev. *Drug Metabolism Drug Interaction* 4 (1983): 339.

Howell, Edward. *Enzyme Nutrition*. (Wayne, NJ: Avery, 1985.)

Hunter, Beatrice Trum. *How Safe Is Food in Your Kitchen?* (New York: Scribner's, 1981.)

————. *Gluten Intolerance: The Widespread Genetic Defect That Can Cause Arthritis, Enteritis, Schizophrenia and Other Health Problems.* (New Canaan, CT: Keats Publishing, Inc., 1987.)

Jacques, P. F. "Effect of vitamin C on HDL and blood pressure." *Journal of the American College of Nutrition* 9(5) (1990): 554/Abstract 106.

Jenkins, D. J. A., T. M. S. Woelver, and R. H. Taylor. "Glycemic index of foods: A physiological basis for carbohydrate exchange." *American Journal of Clinical Nutrition* 34 (1981): 362–66.

Jones, Jeanne. *Food Lovers Diet.* (San Francisco: 101 Productions, 1982.)

Kalyana, S. "Replacement of dietary fat with palm oil; effect on human serum lipids, lipoproteins and apoliproteins." *British Journal of Nutrition* 68 (1992): 677–92.

Kaplan, N. "The deadly quartet: upper body obesity, glucose intolerance, hypertriglyceridemia and hypertension." *Archives of Internal Medicine* 149 (1989): 1514–20.

Kinderlehrer, J. "B6—Maybe the answer to heart disease." *Prevention,* September 1979: 138.

Kinsella, J. E., et al. "Metabolism of trans fatty acids with emphasis on the effect trans, trans-octadecadienoate on lipid composition, essential fatty acid, and prostaglandins; an overview." *American Journal of Clinical Nutrition* 34 (1981): 2307–18.

Kozlovsky, A., et al. "Effects of diets high in simple sugars on urinary chromium losses." *Metabolism* 35 (6) (1986): 515–18.

Kremer, J. M., et al. "Effects of manipulation of dietary fatty acids on clinical manifestations of rheumatoid arthritis." *Lancet* 184 (1985).

Kuczmarski, Robert J., Dr. PH, R.D., et al. "Increasing prevalence of overweight among US adults." *Journal of the American Medical Association* 3 (1994): 205–11.

Kugler, Hans, M.D. *Dr. Kugler's Seven Keys to a Longer Life.* (New York: Stein and Day, 1978.)

Kummerow, F. A., et al. "Saturated Fat and Cholesterol: Dietary

'Risk-Factors' or Essentials to Human Life?" *Food and Nutrition News,* September-October 1981.

———. "Nutrition imbalance and angiotoxins as dietary risk factors in coronary heart disease." *American Journal of Clinical Nutrition* 32 (1979): 58–83.

Lau, B., et al. "Allium (Garlic) and Atherosclerosis: A Review." *Nutrition Research* 3 (1983): 119.

Lecos, C. "Safety Tips for the Outdoor Chef." *Health Connections Magazine,* July 1985: 8.

Lee, Tak. H., et al. "Effect of dietary enrichment with Icosapentaenoic and Dicosahexaenoic acids on in vitro neutrophil and monocyte leukotriene generation and neutrophil function." *New England Journal of Medicine* 312 (1985): 1217.

Lefavi, Robert G., Ph.D. "Has chromium been overlooked as a hypolipidemic agent?" *The Nutrition Report* 9(9), September 1991: 65–72.

Lipetz, Philip, Ph.D. *The Good Calorie Diet.* (New York: HarperCollins, 1994.)

Lovell, C. R., et al. "Treatment of Atopic Eczema with Evening Primrose Oil." *Lancet* 278 (1981).

Lyinsky, W., et al. "Benzo-pyrene and other polynuclear hydrocarbons in charbroiled meat." *Science* 145 (1985): 2.

Mann, John A. *Secrets of Life Extension.* (Berkeley: And/or Press, 1980.)

May, John. *Curious Facts.* (New York: Holt, Rinehart and Winston, 1980.)

McCully, K., et al. "Production of Arteriosclerosis by Homocysteinemia." *American Journal of Pathology* 61, no. 1 (1970): 1.

Mensink, R. P., and M. B. Katan. "Effect of dietary trans fatty acids on high density and low density lipoprotein cholesterol levels in healthy subjects." *New England Journal of Medicine* 323 (1990): 439–45.

Mertz, Walter. "Chromium in human nutrition: a review." *American Institute of Nutrition* 123 (1993): 626–30.

"Obesity Linked to Metabolism in Brown Fat." *Chemical Engineering News,* February 16, 1981: 25.

O'Neill, Molly. "So It May Be True After All: Eating Pasta Makes You Fat." *New York Times,* February 8, 1995: A1 and C6.

Olefsky, J. M., et al. "Effects of weight reduction on obesity:

studies of carbohydrate and lipid metabolism." *Journal of Clinical Investigation* 53 (1974): 64–76.

Ornish, Dean, M.D. *Stress, Diet, and Your Heart.* (New York: Holt, Rinehart and Winston, 1983.)

Oski, Frank, M.D. *Don't Drink Your Milk.* (Syracuse, NY: Mollica Press, Ltd., 1983.)

Oster, K. "Predisposition to atherosclerosis" letter. *Journal of the American Medical Association* 222 (1972): 704.

Oster, Kurt A., M.D., and Donald J. Ross, Ph.D. *Homogenized Milk May Cause Your Heart Attack: The XO Factor.* (New York: Park City Press, 1983.)

Ott, John N. *Health and Light.* (New York: Pocket Books, 1976.)

Page, Melvin, D.D.S. *Chemistry in Health and Disease.* (La Mesa, CA: Price Pottenger Foundation Reprint, 1984.)

Passwater, Richard, Ph.D. *Evening Primrose Oil.* New Canaan, CT: Keats Publishing, 1981.)

Pearce, M., et al. "Incidence of cancer in men on a diet high in polyunsaturated fat." *Lancet* 464 (1971).

Pennington, Jean A. T., and Helen Nichols Church. *Bowes and Church's Food Values of Portions Commonly Used.* (Philadelphia: J. B. Lippincott Company, 1985.)

Phillipson, B., and William E. Connor, et al. "Reduction of plasma lipids, lipoproteins, and apoproteins by dietary fish oils in patients with hypertriglyceridemia." *New England Journal of Medicine* 312 (1985): 1210.

Pinckney, Edward, M.D., and D. Pinckney. *The Cholesterol Controversy.* (Los Angeles: Sherbourne Press, Inc., 1973.)

———. "The potential toxicity of excessive polyunsaturates." *American Heart Journal* 85 (1973): 723.

Pritikin, Nathan, with J. Patrick McCrady. *The Pritikin Program for Diet and Exercise.* (New York: Grosset and Dunlap, 1979.)

Raloff, J. "Oxidized lipids: a key to heart disease." *Science News* 129:278.

———. "Reason for boning up on manganese." *Science News,* September 27, 1986.

Randolph, Theron, G., M.D., and Ralph W. Moss, Ph.D. *An Alternative Approach to Allergies.* (New York: Bantam, 1981.)

Reaven, G. "Role of abnormalities of carbohydrate and lipoprotein metabolism in the pathogenesis and clinical course of hypertension." *Journal of Cardiovascular Pharmacology* 15 (supp5) (1990): S4–7.

———. "Role of insulin resistance in human disease." *Diabetes* 37 (1988): 595–607.

Rendelman, R. "Dr. Edward Howell: A man with an urgent message." *Bestways Magazine,* May 1979, reprint.

Rinkel, H. J. "Food allergy: The role of food allergy in internal medicine." *Annals Allergy* 2 (1944): 115–24.

Roberts, H. J. *Sweet'ner Dearest: Bittersweet Vignettes About Aspartame (NutriSweet).* (West Palm Beach: Sunshine Sentinel Press, 1992.)

———. *Aspartame (NutriSweet): Is It Safe?* (Philadelphia: The Charles Press, 1989.)

Rosenvold, Lloyd, M.D. *Can a Gluten-Free Diet Help You . . . How?* (New Canaan, Ct: Keats Publishing, Inc., 1992.)

Rowe, A. H. *Food Allergy, Its Manifestations, Diagnosis and Treatment.* (Philadelphia: 1983.)

Rudin, D. "The major psychoses and neurosis as Omega-3 essential fatty acid deficiency syndrome: Substrate beriberi." *Med. Hypotheses* 8 (1982): 17.

Schroeder, Henry A. *The Poisons Around Us.* (Bloomington, IN: Indiana University Press, 1974.)

Sears, Barry, Ph.D. "Essential fatty acids and dietary endocrinology: a hypothesis for cardiovascular treatment." *Journal of Advancement in Medicine* 6 (winter 1993): 4211–24.

Shurkin, Joel. "Artificial sweeteners." *Healthline,* October 1983:10.

Siguel, Edward N., M.D., Ph.D. *Essential Fatty Acids in Health and Disease.* (Brookline: Nutrek Press, 1994.)

Simonoff, Monique. "Chromium deficiency and cardiovascular risk." *Cardiovascular Research* 18 (1984): 591–96.

Stout, R. "Insulin and atheroma—an update." *Lancet* (1987): 1077–79.

Taub, Harald J. *Keeping Healthy in a Polluted World.* (New York: Harper & Row, 1974.)

Taylor, C. B., et al. "Spontaneously occurring angiotoxic derivatives of cholesterol." *American Journal of Clinical Nutrition* 32 (1979): 40.

Thomas, L. "Mortality from arteriosclerotic disease and consumption of hydrogenated oils and fats." *Brit. J. Preven. Soc. Med.* 29 (1975): 82.

Thomas, L. H. "Hydrogenated oils and fats: the presence of chemically modified fatty acids in human adipose tissue." *American Journal of Clinical Nutrition* 34 (1981): 877–86.

Toufexis, A. "Dieting: the Losing Game." *Time,* January 20, 1986:54.

Truss, C. Orian. *The Missing Diagnosis.* (Birmingham, AL: P.O. Box 26508, Birmingham, 35226. 1983.)

———. "The Role of Candida Albicans in Human Illness." *Journal of Orthomolecular Psychiatry* 10, no. 4 (1981).

Urberg, Martin, M.D., et al. "Hypocholesterolemic effects of nicotemic acid and chromium supplementation." *The Journal of Family Practice* 27 (1988): 6.

U.S. Department of Agriculture. *Composition of Foods, Fats and Oils, Raw, Processed, Prepared.* USDA Agricultural Handbook No. 8–4, 1979.

U.S. Department of Health, Education and Welfare. *Healthy People: The Surgeon General's Report on Health Promotion and Disease Prevention.* (Washington, DC: Government Printing Office, 1979.)

U.S. Senate Select Committee on Nutrition and Human Needs. *Dietary Goals for the United States.* Second edition. (Washington, DC: Government Printing Office, 1977.)

Vaddadi, K. S., and D. F. Horrobin. "Weight loss produced by evening primrose oil administration in normal and schizophrenic individuals." *IRCS Medical Science* (1979): 52.

Willet, C. W., et al. "Intake of trans fatty acid and risk of coronary heart disease among women." *Lancet* 341 (1993): 581–85.

Willet, C. W., and A. Ascherio. "Trans fatty acids: are the effects only marginal?" *American Journal of Public Health* 84 (May 1994): 722–24.

Woelver, T. M. S. "Relationship between dietary fiber content and composition in foods and the glycemic index." *American Journal of Clinical Nutrition* 51 (1990): 72–75.

Wurtman, Richard J. "The effects of light on the human body." *Scientific American* 233, no. 1 (July 1975): 68–77.

Yudkin, J. *Sweet and Dangerous.* (New York: Bantam Books, 1974.)

Zavaroni, Ivana, M.D., et al. "Risk factors for coronary artery disease in healthy persons with hyperinsulinemia and normal glucose tolerance." *New England Journal of Medicine* 320 (1989): 702–6.

Zock, P. L., and M. B. Katan. "Hydrogenation alternatives: effects of trans fatty acids and stearic acid versus linoleic acid on serum lipids and lipoproteins in humans." *Journal of Lipid Research* 33 (1992): 1493–1501.

RECIPE INDEX

Apple, baked, 218
Applesauce, 218–19
Artichoke omelet, 210–11

Beef
  brisket of beef dinner, 206–207
  Mediterranean meatballs, 203–204
  stuffed peppers oreganato, 205
Black bean soup, 199
Blueberry banana sorbet, 223
Bombay curry sauce, 194
Brisket of beef dinner, 206–207

Cajun cod, 202–203
Carob gelatin, 222
Carrots and snow peas, minted, 216
Cherry gelatin, 221–22
Chicken
  with sherry dijon, 203
  and vegetable sauté, five spice, 207–208
Chickpea sesame pâté, 196–97
Chili mayonnaise, 195
Coconut rum pudding, 220
Coleslaw, 216–17
Cranberry juice, 175

Desserts. See Fruit; Gelatins; Puddings; Sorbets
Dressings, Salad. See Salad dressings and sauces

Eggs
  artichoke omelet, 210–11
  spinach fritatta, 211
Equivalents, food, 224–31
Eskimo salad niçoise, 207

Fish
  Cajun cod, 202–203
  halibut, lemon-baked, 205
  halibut shrimp kabob, 210
  salmon, baked in wine, 208
  salmon croquettes, 204
  salmon loaf, spiced, 208–209
  tuna, grilled, 209
French olive oil dressing, 192–93

Fruit
  apple, baked, 215
  applesauce, 218–19
  pears, vanilla, 218
  rhubarb sauce, 219
  see also Gelatins; Sorbets
Fruit compote pudding, 221

Garlic roasted peppers and anchovies, 215–16
Gazpacho, 200–201
Gelatins
  carob, 222
  cherry, 221–22
  piña colada, 222
  pomegranate, 222
Ginger pear sorbet, 223
Grain recipe, basic, 224
Greek lentil soup, 199–200

Halibut, lemon-baked, 205
Halibut shrimp kabob, 210
Hazelnut dressing, 191–92
Hollandaise, 195–96
Horseradish sauce with dill, 196

Jack's party pâté, 197–98

Long Life Cocktail, 174

Maple pudding, 220–21
Mediterranean meatballs, 203–204
Muffin, magic, 219–20

Pâtés
  chickpea sesame pâté, 196–97
  Jack's party pâté, 197–98
  sweetheart pâté, 198
Peanut dressing with ginger and garlic, 193
Pears, vanilla, 218
Peppers and anchovies, garlic roasted, 215–16
Peppers oreganato, stuffed, 205
Pesto, 194
Piña colada gelatin, 222

Pomegranate gelatin, 222
Poultry. *See* Chicken
Puddings
    coconut rum, 220
    fruit compote, 221
    maple, 220–21
    tapioca, 221

Ratatouille, 215
Rhubarb sauce, 219

Safflower dressing with papaya and
        tarragon, 192
Salad dressings and sauces
    Bombay curry sauce, 194
    chili mayonnaise, 195
    French olive oil dressing, 192–93
    fresh tomato piquant, 194–95
    hazelnut dressing, 191–92
    herbed hollandaise, 195–96
    horseradish sauce, 196
    peanut dressing, 193
    Perfect Pesto, 194
    safflower dressing, 192
    sesame lemon dressing, 193
    walnut raspberry vinaigrette, 192
Salads
    coleslaw, 216–17
    Eskimo salad niçoise, 207
Salmon croquettes, 204
Salmon in wine, baked, 208
Salmon loaf, spiced, 208–209

Sauces. *See* Salad dressings and
        sauces
Sesame lemon dressing, 193
Sorbets
    blueberry banana, 223
    ginger pear, 223
Soups
    black bean, sherried, 199
    gazpacho, 200–201
    Greek lentil, 199–200
    split pea and yam, 201
    vegetable bean, 201–202
Spinach fritatta, 211
Split pea and yam soup, 201
Substitutions, 231–32
Sweetheart pâté, 198

Tapioca, 221
Tomato piquant, 194–95
Tuna, grilled, 209

Vegetable bean soup, 201–202
Vegetables
    carrots and snow peas, minted, 216
    peppers and anchovies, garlic
        roasted, 215–16
    ratatouille, 215
    see also Salads

Walnut raspberry vinaigrette, 192

Yam and split pea soup, 201
Yogurt cheese, 164

INDEX

Adrenal glands, 102
Aerobic exercise, 34, 97, 108–12, 115, 176
Agar-agar, 149
Airplane meals, 241
ALA (alpha-linolenic acid), 89, 90
Alcohol, 85, 115, 165–66
  organic, sources of, 152, 157
  recommended types and brands, 149
Allergies, 7, 19, 134
Allicin, 94
Almond oil, 113
  recommended brands, 141
Aluminum, 133
Alzheimer's disease, 24, 133
Amaranth, 224
Amazing Facts, 69
Amenorrhea, 7
American Heart Association, 28, 80, 241
American Journal of Cardiology, 63
American Journal of Nutrition, 78
American Physician Family Journal, The, 168
American Soybean Association, 71
Anderson, James, 105
Anderson Hospital and Tumor Institute, 94
Anemia, 80
Angostura bitters, 232
Antacids, 133
Antioxidants, 42, 93
Apples, 125
Arachidonic acid, 57
Archer, Douglas, 118
Arthritis, 19, 21, 56
Ascriptin, aluminum in, 133
Ascherio, Alberto, 63
Aspartame, 98, 148
Aspergillus niger, 94
Asthma, 21
Atkins, Robert, 4
Avidin, 127
Avocado oil, 66

Baking, 128
Baking powder, recommended brands, 146
Baking soda
  sodium in, 137
  vitamin destruction, 117
Bang, H. O., 14
Bantus, 14
Beans, 105, 127
  organic, suppliers of, 151, 152, 153, 155, 156, 157, 158, 159
  recommended types, 147
  seasoning for, 235
  storage, 147
Beef, 144
  organic suppliers of, 153, 154, 157, 160
  See also Recipe Index
Beef tallow, 69, 116
Beta carotene, 42, 93, 115
Beverages, 148
  see also specific beverage
Beyond Pritikin Diet
  Eleven Point Prescription, 170–71
  Fat Flush program, 173–79
  fats, 17–18, 87–92
  Master Formula, 33, 181–82
  Master Menu Plan, 3, 169, 182–91
  nutritional discoveries, 117
  questions about, 162–70
  recipes. *See* Recipe Index
  recommended foods and brands, 141–49
  restaurant and travel trips, 237–42
  transitional tips, 231–32
  weight loss on, 29–30, 168–69
Bicycling, 111–12
Bieler, Henry, 81–83
Bile, 73, 104
Bio Foods, Inc., 6
Biosocial Publications International, 246
Blackberries, 125
Blackburn, George, 70
Black currant oil, 88
Blueberries, 125

Borage, 16, 88
Bordia, Arun, 96
Boston University Medical Center, 17
Bowel disorders, 104, 134
Brain disorders, 57
Brains (food), 88
Bran, oat, 104, 105, 232
Breads
  organic, suppliers of, 154, 155, 156,
    157, 159, 160
  recommended brands and storage,
    146
Breast-feeding, 90–91
Brine, 137
Brody, Jane, 26
Broiling, 128
Bufferin, aluminum in, 133
Burger King, 73
Burkitt, Denis, 106
Business Trend Analysts, Inc., 74
Butter, 8, 78, 169

Caffeine, 102
Cajun spices, supplier of, 236
Calcium, 25, 39, 43–44, 133
Calloway, Wayne, 4
Calories, fat percentage list, 50–51
Can a Gluten-Free Diet Help You . . .
    How?, 24
Cancer, 80
  breast, 95
  colon, 26, 104
  cooking methods related to, 130
  diet and, 22
  essential fat inhibition of, 19
  fish oils in prevention of, 55
  garlic oil to inhibit, 94
  indoles against, 93
  low cholesterol and, 66
Candida albicans, 19, 27, 94, 137
Canning, 117, 120
Canola oil, 67–68, 90
The Carbohydrate Addict's Diet, 4
The Carbohydrate Cravers' Diet, 26
Carbohydrates, 1–12
  absorption, 39
  addiction, 4
  complex, 23
  exchange list, 228–30
  refined, 85
  toxicity, 4
  and women, 7
Cardiovascular disease, 5, 17, 63, 69,
    102
  aerobic exercise to prevent, 109
  fish oil and, 21, 55
  French diet and, 69
  heat-damaged oils and, 78

and serum cholesterol, 14, 18,
    80–81
Carpaccio, 125
Caveman's Diet, 25
Celiac disease. See Gluten, intolerance
Cell membranes, 38
Cellulite, 100
Center for Genetics Nutrition and
    Health, 5
Center for Science in the Public Inter-
    est (CPSI), 70
Cereals, 181–82
  organic, suppliers of, 154, 155, 156,
    157, 158
  recommended brands, 145
Charcoal grilling, 130
Cheese, 115, 153, 160
Chewing food, 139
Chicken. See Poultry; Recipe Index
Chinese food, 240
Cholesterol
  and cardiovascular disease, 14, 18,
    79–84
  function, 77
  level in blood, 79–81, 82–83
  lipoproteins and, 79
  oxidation of, 78, 115
  serum, 14, 18, 32
  sources, 58–59, 78
  stress and, 80
Choline, 98, 100
Chopping boards, 118, 132
Chromium, 7, 98–99
Cigarettes. See Tobacco
Cis fatty acids, 40, 42
Clorox, 123, 132
  cleansing formula, 149–51
Coconut oil, 69–73, 88, 113, 116
Coffee, 85, 164–65
  decaffeinated, 165
  substitutes, 148
Colon cancer, 26, 104
Community Nutrition Institute, 64
Condiments, 147
Connor, William, 18
Constipation, 26
Convenience foods, 74
  see also Fast foods
Cooking, 117, 119, 120
  fish, fowl, and meat, 125–26
  fruit, 124–25
  recommended methods and uten-
    sils, 127–29, 131–34
  seeds, peanuts, nuts, beans, egg
    whites and potatoes, 127
  undesirable methods and utensils,
    129–31, 132–34
  vegetables, 124

Cookware. *See* Utensils, cooking; types
Copper cookware, 133
Corning Ware, 131
Corn oil, 88
    recommended brands, 141
Cottonseed oil, 73, 88, 136
Crackers, recommended brands, 145
Cranberry juice, 33, 175
Cranberry sauce, 232
Crayhorn, Robert, 95
Crisco, 62
Crook, William, 26
Cryptosporidium, 134
Cutting boards, 118, 132

Dairy products
    exchange list, 231
    on *Beyond Pritikin* Diet, 163–64
    recommended brands, 142–43
    storage, 143
    see also specific product
Dairy tin bakeware, 134
Dancing, 111
Death, causes of, 46–47
Deodorants, 133
Department of Health and Human Sci-
        ences, 46
Depression, 25
Detoxification, 175–77
DHA (docosahexaenoic acid), 15
Diabetes, 5, 19, 22, 49, 55, 64, 80, 95,
        102, 106
Diarrhea, 134
Dietary Goals for the United States, 22
Dietary supplements, 91, 114–15, 166–
        68, 174–75
Diet for a Small Planet, 25
Diets
    fad, 46
    high carbohydrate, 23–24
    see also Beyond Pritikin Diet; Priti-
        kin Nutrition Program
Di-Gel, aluminum in, 133
Digestion, 139–40
Docosahexaenoic acid. *See* DHA
Down's syndrome, 24
Dr. Atkins' New Diet Revolution, 4
Drugs and drug products. *See* medi-
        cations; specific kinds
Dry eye, 57
Dryerberg, John, 14–15

Educational resources, 243–47
Eggs
    avidin in, 127
    cholesterol and cooking method,
        78–79
    Clorox bath for, 150–51

dried, 115
    enzyme inhibitors in, 127
    seasoning for, 235
    see also Recipe Index
Eicosapentaenoic acid. *See* EPA
Eleven-Point Prescription, 170–71
Enamel cookware, 131
Enig, Mary, 64, 71
Enzymatic cofactors, 53
Enzyme Nutrition, 101
EPA (eicosapentaenoic acid), 15, 18,
        52–56, 88–92, 114
Ephedra, 102
Equivalents, food, 224–31
Erasmus, Udo, 18
Eskimos, 15, 55, 101
Essential fats
    benefits of, 8, 18–19
    in *Beyond Pritikin* Diet, 17–18, 31–32
    defined, 60–61
    in Fat Flush program, 32
    necessity for, 17
    prostaglandins, transformation
        into, 53
    sources of, 16–17, 90–92
    see also Omega-3 fatty acids;
        Omega-6 fatty acids
Ethnic dining, 239–41
Evening primrose oil, 16, 47, 88
Exchange lists, 224–31
Exercise plan, 33–34, 108–12, 115
Extracts, flavor, 147
Eye. *See* Retina; Tear production

Fad diets, 46
Fast foods, 69, 73, 78
Fat, body
    brown, 30–31, 48–49
    white, 30, 48
Fat, dietary
    basic groups, 36–38
    calories, percentage of, 50–51
    in convenience foods, 75
    damaged, 29, 35, 40–43, 83–85, 115
    exchange list, 225
    food label terminology, 135–36
    functions of, 38–40
    monounsaturated, 37, 66–67
    in Pritikin diet, 14, 15, 18, 19–20
    saturated, 37, 73, 81, 116
    see also Essential fats; GLA; Omega-
        3 fatty acids; Omega-6 fatty acids;
        Polyunsaturated fats
Fat Flush program, 8, 32, 173–79
FDA (Food and Drug Administration),
        3, 118
Felix Letter, The, 247

Fermented foods, 26
Fiber, 32, 74, 103–107, 114
Fingernails, 19, 23
Fish
  canned, 143
  Clorox bath for, 151
  cooking and storing, 125–26
  raw, 125
  recommended types, 114, 143
  seasoning for, 234
  shellfish, 126–27, 143
  see also Oils, fish; Recipe Index
Fish Oil. See Oils, fish
Flavor extracts, 147
Flaxseed, 53, 89–90, 142, 231
Flaxseed oil, 8, 57, 61, 113
Flours, 146
  organic, suppliers of, 151, 154, 156,
    157, 158
Foil, aluminum, 133
Folic acid, 24
"Food Guide Pyramid," 2, 3, 20
Food Is Your Best Medicine, 82
Food poisoning, 118
Food preparation and storage, 116–34
Food Values of Portions Commonly
  Used, 167
Fowl. See Poultry
Free radicals, 42, 79, 93
Freezing, 117, 120
French food, 240
Friedman, Meyer, 80
Frozen dinners, 74–75
Fruit
  on Beyond Pritikin Diet, 162–63
  citrus, 93
  Clorox bath for, 151
  exchange list, 227–28
  exotic, 217
  on Fat Flush program, 174
  fiber source, 105
  juice, 86
  organic, suppliers of, 151–60
  preparation and cooking, 124–25
  preserves, 144–45
  recommended, 114, 144–45
  seasoning for, 236
  selection and storage, 121–22,
    123–24
  sugar source, 86
  see also specific fruit; Recipe Index
Frying, 129–30
Full-spectrum light, 33, 110, 111

Gamma linolenic acid. See GLA
Garlic, 94–96
  organic, suppliers of, 151, 160

Gas stoves, 130
Gelatin, 149
Gelusil, aluminum in, 133
George Washington University, 4
Giardia lamblia, 134
GLA (gamma linolenic acid)
  cis-linolenic acid conversion, 49
  prostaglandin component, 52–54
  sources, 15, 18, 53, 88
  supplements, 92, 114
  treatment with, 28
Glass cookware, 131
Glucagon, 7
Gluten
  grains containing, 23
  grains without, 26
  intolerance, 2, 23–24, 25, 107
Glycemic Index, 6, 8–12, 97, 138,
  171, 174, 182
Goat's milk, 231
Gooseberry oil, 88
Grains
  basic recipe, 224
  exotic, 224
  fiber content, 104
  gluten-free, 26
  organic, suppliers of, 151–60
  recommended types and brands,
    145
  soaking, 127
  storage, 145
  whole, 23–24, 93, 114
Greek food, 240–41
Grilling, 130
Grundy, Scott M., 67
Guarana, 102
Gurewich, Victor, 96

Harvard Medical School, 21
Hazelnut oil, 113
  recommended brands, 141
HDL (high-density lipoproteins), 79, 99
Health and Healing, 70
Health food stores, 138–39
Heart disease. See Cardiovascular dis-
  ease
Heat processing, 40, 49
Heimlich, Jane, 70
Heller, Rachel, 4
Heller, Richard, 4
Herbs, 102, 147, 233–36
  organic, suppliers of, 152, 153, 154,
    157, 158, 159
Hoffman-LaRoche, 15
Homogenization, 42–44, 50, 115
Horrobin, David, 15, 18
Horseradish, 232

Howell, Edward, 101
Hydrogenation, 41, 49, 61–64
Hydroponics, 122
Hypercholestremia, 82
Hypertension, 5, 22, 25, 102
Hypoglycemia, 97

Immune system, 19
Indian food, 241
Indoles, 93
Insotol, 98, 100–101
Insulin, 3–4, 7, 64, 97, 98
Iron, 25, 131–32
Irradiated food, 160–61
Italian food, 239

Jenkins, David, 6
Jogging. See Running
Journal of the American Medical Association, 79, 109
Juice, fruit, 86
  see also Cranberry juice

Kentucky Medical Center, 105
Kidneys (food), 88
Kidney disease, 102
Kola nut, 102
Kummerow, Fred, 63

Labels, food, 135–38
Lamb, 144
Lancet, 15, 63
Lappe, Frances Moore, 25
Lard, 73
L-carnitine, 98, 99–100
LDL (low-density lipoproteins), 79, 99, 100
Legumes. See Beans; Lentils; Peas
Lentils, 105
Light, full-spectrum, 33, 110, 111
Lipase, 98, 101
Lipid Research Clinic's Coronary Primary Prevention Trial, 79–80
Lipids, 36
Lipoproteins, 79
Lipotropics, 100, 101
Live Longer Now, 22
Liver (food), 88
Liver disease, 80, 85
Living the High Carbohydrate Way, 26
Long Life Cocktail, 32, 174
Lucite, 132
Lysine, 100, 224

Maalox, aluminum in, 133
Mademoiselle (magazine), 74
Magnesium, 53, 115

Manganese, 44
Margarine, 61–65, 115, 242
Master Formula, 33, 181–82
Master Menu Plan, 8, 32–33, 169, 182–92
mate, 102
Mayonnaise, 142
Mazola oil, 78
McCully, Kilmer, 93
McDonald's, 69, 73
McDougall, John, 2
McManus, Bruce, 81
MCTs. See Triglycerides
Meat
  Clorox bath for, 151
  food poisoning from, 118
  lean red, 88
  organic sources of, 153, 154, 156, 157, 159, 160
  preparation and storage, 125–26
  raw, 125
  seasoning for, 235
  see also specific meat
Meat and poultry hotline, 126
Medications, 133, 167
  see also specific brand names
Menstruation. See PMS
Menus, 183–91
  see also Recipe Index
Metabolism, 7, 17, 34, 46, 83, 87, 102, 109
Metamucil, 174
Methionine, 100
Mexican food, 240
Microwave, 128–29
Milk, 43–44, 78, 90–91, 115, 119, 231, 232
Mineral oil, 136
Minerals. See Dietary supplements; specific mineral
MIT, 26
Mitochondria, 99
Monounsaturated fats, 37, 66–68
Mount Sinai Hospital, 4
MSG (monosodium glutamate), 137
Multiple sclerosis, 56
Myelin, 38
Mylanta, aluminum in, 133
Myasthenia gravis, 24

National Academy of Sciences, 22, 99
National Heart, Lung and Blood Institute, 81
National Heart Saver Association, 72
National Institutes of Health, 5
New England Journal of Medicine, 21, 67

Newsletters, 244–47
The New York Times, 4
Niacin. *See* Vitamins, B-3
NordicTrack, 110
Nursing. *See* Breast-feeding
Nuts, 38, 88, 127
  organic, sources of, 152, 153, 156, 158
  recommended types, 142
  storage, 142

Oat bran, 104, 105–106, 232
Obesity, 5, 45, 46–47, 49, 64, 81, 99
  see also Weight loss
Oils, fish
  capsules, 92
  and cardiovascular disease, 21, 55, 57
  EPA content of, 89
  in Eskimo diet, 15
  see also Omega headings
Oils, vegetable
  chemical extraction, 59, 60
  cold pressed, 59–60, 66
  crude, 60
  early production methods, 59
  expeller pressed, 60, 113
  in fast foods, 69–70, 73
  on Fat Flush program, 173, 179
  heat-damaged, 78
  monounsaturated, 66–67
  polyunsaturated, 58–65, 69
  processed, 49, 58, 60
  recommended, 113, 141
  saturated, 68–69
  storage, 142
  unprocessed, 88, 113
  see also specific oil
Oleo. *See* Margarine
Olive oil, 8, 66–67, 88, 113
  recommended brands, 114
Omega-3 fatty acids
  DHA (docosahexaenoic acid), 15
  disease treatment with, 28, 57
  EPA (eicosapentaenoic acid), 15, 18, 52–53, 88–89
  prostaglandin formation, 16, 31
  sources, 16, 37, 88–90
  supplements, 92
Omega-6 fatty acids
  disease treatment with, 28, 57
  prostaglandin formation, 16, 31
  sources, 16, 37–38, 61, 90
  supplements, 92
  see also GLA
Onions, 96
  organic, supplier of, 160

Oregon Health Sciences University, 21
Organic food suppliers, 151–60
Organic Merchants Association, 58
Ornish, Dean, 2, 80
Osteoporosis, 43–44
Oster, Kurt A., 43
Oxidation, 41–42, 50, 78, 79, 115

Pabirin, aluminum in, 133
Pain relievers, 133
Palm kernel oil, 68, 69, 116
Palm oil, 68, 69, 72, 116
Parasites, 71, 95, 125
Parcells, Hazel, 149
Parchment paper, cooking in, 133–34
Pasta, 26
  exchange list, 231
  organic, suppliers of, 151, 156, 158
  recommended brands, 146
PCBs (polychlorinated biphenyls), 92
Peanut oil, 66, 67, 88, 113
  recommended brands, 141
Peanuts, 127
Peas, dried, 105
Pesticides, 150
Pierson, Herbert F., 95
PMS (premenstrual syndrome), 7, 19
Pollution, environmental, 93, 167
Polysystemic chronic candidiasis, 27
Polyunsaturated fats
  dangers of, 28, 84–85
  processing of, 58–65
  sources, 37–38
Potatoes, 122, 123, 126, 128, 153–54, 154
  Clorox bath for, 151
  cooking and storage, 125–26
  organic, suppliers of, 154
  recommended types and brands, 143
  salmonella infection of, 118
  seasoning for, 235
Powter, Susan, 2
Premenstrual syndrome. *See* PMS
Preserves, fruit, 144–45
Pressure cooking, 131
Preventive Nutrition Consultants, Inc., 95
Price Pottenger Nutrition Foundation, 245
Pritikin, Nathan
  death of, 21
  fat content of diet, 14, 15, 16–17, 19, 20, 25, 34
  personal health, 13–14
  research, 14–15
Pritikin Longevity Centers, 21

Pritikin Nutrition Program
basics of, 13–14
disadvantages, 23–27
successes, 22
Pritikin Program for Diet and Exercise, The, 15
Procter & Gamble, 62
Prostaglandins
benefits of, 54–57
function of, 16, 52
inflammatory, 55–56, 67, 83
production of, 39, 53–54, 57
Protein
exchange list, 225–26
on Fat Flush program, 173
recommended sources, 143–44
Psoriasis, 25
Publications, nutrition, 244–47
Puka Puka, 70
Puritan oil, 78
Pyrex cookware, 131, 134

Quinoa, 224

Reading, Chris, 25
Reaven, Gerald, 5
Recipes. *See* Recipe Index
Refrigeration, 119–21
Restaurant dining, 237–42
Retina, 33
Riboflavin. *See* Vitamins, B-2
Robert Crayhon's Nutrition Made Simple, 95
Rolaids, aluminum in, 133
Rosenvold, Lloyd, 24
Royal Prestige Cookware, 132
Rudin, Donald, 18
Running, 109–10

SAD (seasonal affective disorder), 111
Safflower oil, 8, 48, 61, 88, 113
recommended brands, 141
Salicylate, 102
S-allylcysteine, 95
Salt, 136–37
recommended types and brands, 148
Saltman, Paul, 44
Saturated fats, 37, 73, 81, 116
Sautéing, 127–28
Sears, Barry, 4, 6, 18
Seasonings. *See* Herbs; Spices
Seeds
ALA source, 38, 90
enzyme inhibitors in, 127

organic, suppliers of, 152, 154, 155, 156, 158
recommended types, 142
storage, 142
Selenium, 42, 49, 93, 96, 115
Senate Select Committee on Nutrition and Human Needs, 22
Sesame oil, 88, 113
recommended brands, 141
Shellfish, 126–27, 143
Shipboard meals, 241
Shopping, 138–39
Shortening, 61, 116
Siguel, Edward, 2, 17, 18
Simopoulos, Artemis P., 4
Skin diseases, 19, 56
Smoking. *See* Tobacco
Sodium, 136–37, 163
Soft drinks, 166
Sokolof, Paul, 72
Solanine, 122
Soups, 147
seasoning for, 235
see also Recipe Index
Soybean oil, 88, 90
recommended brands, 141
Soy sauce, 137, 231
Spectrum Spread, 65
Spicer, Arnold, 106
Spicer's Hunger Crunchers, 106–107
Spices, 147, 233–36
Organic suppliers of, 154, 156, 158
Spittle, Constance, 93
Sprue disease. *See* Gluten, intolerance
Stainless steel cookware, 131, 134
Stanford University Medical School, 5
Steak tartare, 125
Steaming, 128
timetable for vegetables, 212–15
Stir-fry, 127–28
Stoves, gas, 131
Stress, 80, 81
Stress, Diet and Your Heart, 80
Sugar, 85, 115, 137
Sugar virus, 49
Sunflower oil, 8, 88, 113
recommended brands, 141
Sunglasses, 33–34
Sunlight, 33–34
Surgeon General's Report on Health Promotion and Disease Prevention, 10
Sushi, 125
Swanson, Gloria, 81
Sweetbreads, 88
Sweeteners, 148
Swimming, 111

Tamari, 137
Tarahumara Indians, 14, 23
Taylor, C. B., 78
Tear production, 57
Thermogenic response, 30, 47, 102
Thiamin. *See* Vitamins, B-1
Thickeners, 146–47
Thyroid gland, 80
Toasting, 128
Tobacco, 81, 167
Tofu, 144
Tokelauan, 70
Trans fatty acids
  cis form converted to, 40, 41
  prostaglandin blockers, 63, 85
  sources, 49, 73, 115
Triglycerides, 5, 18, 71, 85–86, 99, 100
Truss, Orian, 26
Tufts University, 96
Twain, Mark, 139

University of Leiden, 21
University of Nebraska Medical Center, 81
University of Texas Health Sciences Center, 67
University of Toronto, 6
U.S. Department of Agriculture, 2, 126
Utensils, cooking, 131–34

Vanquish, aluminum in, 133
Veal, 144
Vegetable oil. *See* Oils, vegetable
Vegetables
  Clorox bath for, 150
  cruciferous, 93
  deep yellow, 93
  exchange list, 226–27
  exotic, 212
  on Fat Flush program, 173–74
  fiber content, 105
  green leafy, 88, 89, 90, 93
  organic, suppliers of, 151–60
  preparation and cooking, 124
  recommended, 114, 144
  seasoning for, 235–36
  selecting and storing, 121–23
  steaming timetable, 212–15
  see also Oils, vegetable; specific vegetable; Recipe Index
Vegetarianism, 25
Vinegars, 148, 157, 159
Vitamins
  A, 25, 39, 56
  B group, 24, 39, 100, 119, 127

B-1 (thiamin), 125, 127
B-2 (riboflavin, 119
B-3 (niacin), 49, 53, 115
B-6, 49, 53, 93, 100, 115
B-12, 24
C, 42, 49, 53, 93, 100, 115
D, 39
E, 25, 39, 42, 49, 79, 93, 115
  fat fighters, 93
  fat soluble, 25, 39
  food storage and preparation, 117, 118–19
K, 39
  see also Dietary supplements

Walking, 110–11
Walnut Acres, 76, 107
  address, 158
  recommended brands, 141, 142, 145, 147
Walnut oil, 88, 90, 113
  recommended brands, 141
Wargovich, Michael J., 94
Water
  on *Beyond Pritikin* Diet, 114
  chlorinated, 167
  contaminated, 134
  on Fat Flush program, 175, 176–77
  filtered, 148
Water filter, 148, 149
Weight loss, 18, 29–30, 47, 49, 168–69
Wheat, 25
  See also Grains
White, Michael, 81
White willow bark, 102
Willet, Walter, 63
Wood chopping board, 132
Worcestershire sauce, 231
Wurtman, Judith, 26

Xanthine oxidase. *See* XO
XO, 43, 44

Yeast
  Aspergillus niger, 94
  brewer's, 98
  Candida albicans, 7, 19, 27, 94, 95, 137
  overgrowth, 2
  foods related to, 26, 137
  systemic infection, 56, 137
Yogurt, 115, 132
Your Body Knows Best, 6

Zinc, 7, 53, 56, 93, 115